THE
ULTIMATE
GUIDE
TO
THREESOMES

THE
ULTIMATE
GUIDE
TO
THREESOMES

BY STELLA HARRIS

CLEiS
PRESS

Published in the United States by Cleis Press, an imprint of Start Midnight, LLC, 221 River Street, Ninth Floor, Hoboken, New Jersey 07030.

Printed in the United States.
Cover design: Jennifer Do
Cover image: Shutterstock
Text design: Frank Wiedemann
First Edition.
10 9 8 7 6 5 4 3 2 1

Trade paper ISBN: 978-1-62778-307-1
E-book ISBN: 978-1-62778-520-4

CONTENTS

INTRODUCTION

In my years working as an intimacy educator and sex coach, one of the most common topics clients and students bring up is threesomes. Due to this popularity, I developed a whole class about threesomes and group sex, and I've written numerous articles on the topic. Still, I continue to hear the questions. That's why I knew it was time for an Ultimate Guide to answer all these questions and guide the curious.

Information about sex and sexuality is easier to find now than ever, but unfortunately that's a mixed blessing. Like with any topic, not all the information available is good information, and some of it is downright toxic. For threesomes in particular, many articles—and even whole books—are cringeworthy. The problem I'm seeing in a lot of the writing about threesomes is that the couple with the fantasy is being centered while the potential third is a quarry to be hunted.

From gamification to objectification, a potential sexual partner is being seen as a means to an end, not as a person with their own needs and interests. There's also terrible advice about how to "talk your partner into" a threesome, and more framing that puts one person's desires above the needs of others.

A threesome can be anything from a hot sexual adventure between three people who just met to a loving expression of intimacy between people who have a triad relationship. But what's essential is that everyone involved is having their needs and desires heard, and everyone feels like they have an equal say in what will and won't happen.

With a bit of know-how and some communication skills, your sexual fantasies can become a reality. But reality is always a bit messier than fantasy, and there are logistics to plan for and feelings to consider.

This book will walk you through everything you need to know to figure out if threesomes are right for you, and if so, how to plan and negotiate the threesome of your dreams. You'll learn about considerations for safety and common pitfalls to watch out for. It will also offer plenty of ways for established players to up their communication game and get even more out of each encounter.

Where does all this threesome knowledge come from? This book is based on extensive reading and research, about threesomes in particular and sex and relationships in general. It is also informed by the hundreds (thousands?) of clients and students I've worked with. I've heard their fears, guided their negotiations, and been privy to the outcome of their encounters. Each of those common fears will be addressed in these pages, as well as many possible happy outcomes.

I've also engaged in countless threesomes and group play scenarios of my own. Many of them were lovely, and some left room for improvement. I've learned from my experiences and my missteps, and that knowledge is collected here.

Who Is This For/Language

This book is for anyone who has ever fantasized about a three-some—whether you want to have one in real life, or want to keep multiperson play part of your fantasy life.

This book is for couples and single folks, and for people of every gender. Every combination of genders and bodies can have a threesome, and this book strives to address them all. To these ends, the language used will be as gender neutral as possible, and you can simply insert yourself and your lovers as you see fit.

Despite these goals, it's impossible to ignore the gendered nature of the way our culture discusses sex in general and three-somes in particular. Far more couples than singles come to my threesome classes or to my office to explore the idea in more depth, and this book reflects those statistics—often speaking to an existing couple wanting to explore with a third. But there are particular sections addressed to solo folks wanting to explore threesomes, and all of the content is relevant to all parties—so while you may be tempted to skip some sections, everything is worth a look.

That said, this is a reference book of sorts, so feel free to skip around as needed. Maybe your worries about jealousy are too overwhelming to read about sexual positions right now—that's okay! You can read about how to combat jealousy first, or maybe read some of the sections about whether threesomes are right for you.

As with most books, different parts will resonate at different times. Maybe you read this before you've ever had a threesome, and the planning sections are what speak to you most. After you have a few threesomes under your belt, maybe tools to commu-nicate and negotiate to better meet your needs are what will stand out. My suggestion would be to read the whole book now, and then flip back to particular sections later on, as different situ-ations come up for you.

This book also uses several terms of art—meaning words or phrases that have a specialized meaning within a particular context or community. If you find yourself confused about how I'm using a word or term, check the glossary in the back of the book it's likely covered there.

And although it's covered in the glossary, I want to define upfront how I'm using the word *negotiation*. Many people jump to the anxiety of a salary negotiation or haggling over the price of a car when they hear "negotiation," giving the word a negative connotation. When used in reference to sex, I mean negotiation as the process by which all parties come to mutually satisfying agreements.

We'll get into all the particulars in chapter 14, but negotiation will come up in most sections of this book, because talking to people about what you want, and hearing what they want, is a vital part of any sexual encounter, threesomes included.

Philosophy

Every author has a point of view, and especially for nonfiction or educational material, I think it's important to be transparent about that.

I tell new clients at the beginning of our coaching sessions that I don't have an agenda. And I mean that in both senses of the term. There isn't a curriculum I expect people to follow. Rather, coaching is all about the goals and needs that people bring into the session. Coaching is customized for each client.

I also don't have an agenda in that I don't have an outcome I'm rooting for. If a couple comes to me to explore the idea of opening a relationship, I'm not invested in what path they choose. I don't think polyamory is better than monogamy, or vice versa.

What I *am* invested in is people knowing all their possible options, and being able to choose what's best for them, free of any outside influence. And that includes pressure from partners or the culture at large.

In addition to knowing all the options, I'm invested in people behaving in a way that is ethical. Towards themselves, their partners, their communities, and anyone else they may engage with.

And here's the thing: ethics are very personal. I have my opinions, and you'll read about many of those in the following pages. But it's not for me to tell you, or anyone, what to do.

It's not uncommon in a coaching session for me to lay out a situation for a client, ask the right questions, and get them to the point where they have to make their own ethical choice. And after reading all the content in this book, you'll have your own choices to make.

Here's where my ethics land, and what I think is important:

▸ I believe people should be treated like people, not like a means to an end.

▸ I believe everyone's wants, needs, and desires should be given equal weight in any interaction.

▸ I believe honesty and transparency are vital when negotiating any relationship or sexual encounter.

▸ I believe people should be given all the information relevant to their decision about how, and if, they'd like to engage.

▸ I believe love takes many forms, and that we benefit from thinking outside the mainstream relationship box.

I've heard plenty of times that people think some kind of trickery is necessary to make threesomes or casual sex happen, and it simply isn't true. There are people out there who want the same things you do, and this book will help you connect with them— in an ethical way.

Personal Stories

Throughout this book I illustrate points with personal stories and anecdotes. In most instances names have been omitted or changed. In a few cases, people wanted their real first names used. Some identifying details have also been changed or omitted in order to preserve everyone's privacy.

1

DEFINITIONS

How Do You Define Sex?

When I teach group classes I ask a lot of questions of the attendees. There's more to being an expert than simply lecturing. In fact, studies have shown that people learn more when they come up with their own answers and solutions. One of the questions I like to ask is, "How do you define sex?"

When I ask this at the beginning of a class, attendees look at me like I'm joking. But as soon as people try to answer, they figure out the complexity. And even if someone comes to an easy answer, it likely doesn't align with the answer of the person they're sitting next to.

When there's enough time, I have people break into small groups to discuss. Just like you remember from elementary school, each group comes up with their own definition, then we share them all with the larger group and discuss. It's always tricky for each group to come up with a working definition they can agree on. And when we come together to share, each group has come up with something different. And you know what? No one is wrong. Defining sex is incredibly personal, and everyone can have their own definition.

Why ask this question? Because defining sex is an important first step before you can negotiate sex with other people. Having different definitions for the same words or acts is one of the most common sexual misunderstandings. It's also one of the quickest ways to cross a boundary or get in trouble.

When coming up with an answer, I encourage as broad a definition as possible—having a broad definition of sex allows you a lot more flexibility when it comes to negotiating play with other people and gives you more options for ways to get needs met.

What definition do you have in your mind right now? Take a minute to think about it. Maybe even write it down.

Does your definition involve penetration? Orgasm? More than one person? The more requirements we have for something to be sex, the more ways there are for something to fall short or feel like a failure.

For example, if your definition of sex is penetration with an erection, what happens if the person with a penis can't get an erection? Or if there's no penis involved at all?

Or if your definition requires an orgasm, or mutual orgasm, and one person can't get there—does that invalidate everything that you and the other person just shared?

We can have orgasms by ourselves. So when we're having sex with other people, it's about more than just getting off. It can be about building or maintaining intimacy and connection. It can be about skin-to-skin contact and the pleasure of touch. It's about exploring—both what other people like, and what we can learn about ourselves in relation to other people.

Maybe sex is pleasure; solo, partnered, or in groups. Maybe sex is an intention to share something intimate. Maybe sex is play. Whatever feels like a good fit for you, try for a broad and flexible definition. And then consider how that definition can include three bodies.

What "Counts" as a Threesome?

So you've just come up with a working definition of sex for yourself. Does that mean that's what a threesome includes? Not necessarily. While you might have a very specific fantasy in mind, having a broad definition of a threesome is just as helpful as having a broad definition of sex.

Especially when it comes to a first threesome—either your first ever, or your first with a particular combination of people—it can be a great idea to start small. There doesn't need to be nudity or genitally focused sex acts for a threesome to be fun.

What about snuggling and watching a movie together? What about a three-way make out? Maybe even a game of strip poker or sexy D&D. A three-way massage session can be a great start. It can involve clothes coming off as well as taking turns as the center of attention. And the communication used for massage can be very similar to the communication used during sex, so it's a great trial run to make sure everyone can use their words, and that everyone is listening.

Maybe you decide to try group massage, and the boundary is that everyone leaves their underwear on—plus no touching over underwear areas. This is a great chance to find out if people are able to respect boundaries in the heat of the moment, or if they get carried away. And that includes whether they continue to ask about doing something that has already been stated as a boundary or limit.

Massage is also a great way to see if the group finds balance in terms of who is giving and who is receiving touch. Does one person always end up the center of attention? Figuring out all these details before everyone is naked can be very helpful.

At some point we seem to reach an age when just making out or flirting doesn't feel like "enough," but I encourage you to give those kinds of encounters a chance. You may be surprised at how hot they can be.

In Justin Lehmiller's book *Tell Me What You Want,* he recounts the results of what, to date, has been the largest survey of sexual fantasies of American adults. And guess what? Of the men and women surveyed, 57.4% and 69.3% respectively report fantasizing about kissing "often." So don't ignore this option!

To do this as an exercise, set a night aside when you'll confine your intimacy within certain parameters. Maybe it's all kissing, maybe there's touching above the waist—the details are up to you. But set boundaries that keep you wanting more.

Now explore what it's like to kiss and touch when it's not just a prelude to something else, but the main event. What are you noticing that you usually miss? Are you more aware of how your partner's lips feel against yours? Are you paying more attention to the noises they make or the way their body moves?

Having a few restrictions can open up a whole new world of exploration and experimentation, because those boundaries force us out of our usual routines.

How else can you expand your thinking as to what "counts" as a threesome?

You may be imagining a threesome as three people in a bed together—but what if one of the participants is on the phone, or on video chat? For many people, this can feel like a safer way to explore the fantasy, and for people with long-distance partners or partners who travel for work, this can be a great way to add some passion and connection between visits. For a first threesome with a particular partner you may want to be in the same place for ease of check-ins and aftercare,[1] but once you know it's something you enjoy, your imagination is the only limit.

---

1   Aftercare is what it sounds like, whatever you need for taking care of yourself after an intense experience. Check out Chapter 24 for more information about aftercare.

Thinking Beyond the Standard

I met a couple from a dating app for a drink, and we all hit it off. The conversation was well rounded, and not just about sex. Everyone took turns talking, and they seemed genuinely interested in me as a person. I was also watching the way they interacted with each other. They both seemed comfortable and confidant, and would occasionally glance at each other to check in.

I asked my usual questions about their level of experience and what they were looking for. They'd played with other couples, in a full swap scenario, but they'd never had a threesome—they were hoping I'd be their first.

In their prior experiences they'd mostly played in the same room, so they were able to see what their partner was up to. This meant they had a pretty good idea of how they felt about sharing, and whether jealousy was a common issue.

The couple were a man and a woman, and the woman didn't have much experience with other women, but she was curious. This can go either way for me, and it really comes down to the person and their attitude.

Back in my teen years, more than one friend came to me with their curiosities. I was open about my sexuality from an early age and that meant people came to me with questions. I was always hesitant to be someone's first same-sex kiss because if they ended up having complicated feelings about it, our friendship would get mixed up in those feelings.

But with a casual play partner or one-off threesome encounter, it can feel safer to be part of someone's exploration. There's no existing relationship to ruin and no shared social circles to complicate.

As our conversation continued, it came out that they were also curious about kink, and rope bondage in particular. It seemed like we were a good fit. After a few more questions about safety and expectations I went back to their place. And after a long snuggle with their adorable puppy we headed to the bedroom. Luckily, I'd recently taught a kink class, so I had my bag of tricks in my car—far more goodies than I'd usually bring on a first date.

We started by just kissing for a long while. Taking turns and feeling each other out. It can take a moment to learn the rhythms of a new person. What level of intensity do they gravitate towards? Do they kiss with urgency or with relaxed sensuality?

Figuring out how the kissing works gives you a lot of clues as to how other activities will flow. Is one person more likely to take charge and make first moves? Is it clear that the people involved enjoy watching as much as participating?

Once we'd built a lot of comfort and the clothes had started coming off, we moved to something the woman was especially interested in: being tied up. Rope bondage requires a lot of communication, especially when you're playing with someone new. So bringing out the rope was a great way to facilitate learning more about her and what she liked, as well as essentials like how her body moves, and if she had any injuries I needed to know about.

Based on her answers to my questions, I tied her in a sensual but playful way, explaining to both of them what I was doing as I was doing it. Together we discovered what she liked about rope and leaned into the things that were working for her. While I was doing the tying, her partner was able to kiss and tease her. Eventually he and I both used hands and fingers on her until she had an orgasm, and then the rope came off.

Next, the man shared something he'd been curious about but hadn't had a chance to try—prostate play. I grabbed some of the lube and gloves from my kit, and we began a slow warm-up. Again, this was both sexy and playful as I described to them what I was doing. Eventually my fingers were inside him, and the look on his face said it all—prostate play was a hit. While I focused on internal pleasure, his partner used her hands and mouth on his penis until he had an orgasm.

From there we snuggled, talked, wound down, and eventually I headed home (though not before snuggling the puppy again). I didn't receive any below the waist contact, and there was never PIV (penis in vagina) sex.

So, does that "count" as a threesome? I sure think so. And to my mind, it incorporated many of the best things a threesome has to offer: being a safe place for people to try things that are brand new, and having the support of their trusted partner right there with them.

I will caution that this is a nonstandard threesome scenario, and you shouldn't count on a third to show up, blow your minds, and leave—but luckily sometimes that's my kink.

The Myth of the Organic Threesome

One of the things I hear most often is that people want a threesome to "just happen." And while once in a blue moon maybe three people fall into bed together without much discussion in advance, I wouldn't recommend it.

What are these potential scenarios in which a spontaneous threesome could happen? Maybe a friend is over for dinner and you try to move things in a sexy direction? All too often that's done by making jokes that make everyone uncomfortable, or making a move that's unwanted. And that's a great way to ruin a friendship.

Or maybe you're out at a bar, see someone cute across the room, and suggest some play with you and your partner? Sure, there's a one in one hundred chance that'll work. But far more likely, the person will think you're being creepy. After all, it's hard enough to try standard dating in the wild—looking for something specific is even harder. You can't tell by looking at someone if they're available for dating, or what kind of people they're into, let alone whether they're into multiperson play. Movies and television might make it seem like everyone is game for sex all the time, but that's not how things work in the real world.

When threesomes look organic or spontaneous from the outside, that's usually because there's been a lot of groundwork behind the scenes that you didn't get to see. Or because when friends are telling you about their adventures, they're leaving out some details to make a better story.

It's also worth noting that partners who regularly play with others likely have a lot of standing agreements, allowing for shorthand in the moment. You'll read more about those situations later in the book, especially when it comes to play parties.

One thing that is common among unplanned or supposedly spontaneous threesomes is the inclusion of alcohol or other intoxicants to lower inhibitions—but that can lead to actions that some or all parties may regret later. While a lot of people are in the habit of having a drink to build confidence, if you need to be drunk to do something, it's likely something you're simply not ready to do.

If "organic" or "spontaneous" is shorthand for not talking about it, and not negotiating, here are some things you can miss:

▸ Safer sex agreements.

▸ Language preferences around gender and body parts.

▸ Likes and dislikes.

▸ Relationship agreements.

▸ Ongoing expectations.

When you know the parameters, you can improvise within them. When you don't know what the parameters are, you're just making wild guesses that can miss the mark. So give up the idea of a threesome "just happening." A bit of planning will make for a much better experience for all involved.

Missing the Mark

Years ago, a date and I ended up staying out too late at a kinky play party and our play partner missed their ride home. Not only that, but our kink play had gotten heavier than intended, and I didn't think leaving our play partner alone in the middle of the night was a great idea.

This was our first mistake. We shouldn't have let the play escalate if we didn't already have an aftercare plan in place, and we also shouldn't have been playing with them before knowing how they planned to get home.

Nevertheless, making the best of what we had to work with, I suggested we all go back to my place for some aftercare, and we could address the transportation issue the next day. We piled into my bed and got some decent sleep.

The next morning, I was woken up by the two of them fooling around. There had been no explicit check-ins and our play the night before had been kinky, not sexual, so this was outside of our negotiations. It became clear that they were headed towards hot and heavy and that no talking was going to happen. I had a choice between a "spontaneous" threesome, or getting out of there.

I choose the latter. I headed to the other room, grabbed my laptop, and tried to get some work done, while listening to sex sounds from my bedroom.

Eventually they emerged, and I made breakfast for everyone, and then drove our unexpected guest home.

Later, my date and I had a long talk about what had happened. I explained how uncomfortable it made me to be put in that position, and how much important information was missed because they didn't stop for a conversation.

What Threesomes Are, And Are Not, For

Threesomes are:

- A great way to try something new, with the potential added support of a partner or friend with you.

- A way to share new kinds of intimacy.

- A way to live out fantasies.

- A chance to explore new people, new bodies, or new dynamics.

- An opportunity to see your partner from a new angle.

- A way to celebrate sex and sexuality.

- A way to confront jealousy, and let go of possessiveness.

Threesomes are not:

- A bandage for a troubled relationship.

- A grudging compromise when one partner wants an open relationship and the other doesn't.

- A chance to ignore a third person's feelings, wants, or needs.

- An excuse to bend agreements or boundaries.

- A chance to "test" your partner.

- A solution for boredom.

THREESOMES IN CULTURE

Threesomes on Screen

Threesomes have been a fixture of film and other media for decades, often used as a shorthand way to say certain things about a character—all too often, unsavory things. Or they're used to simply titillate the audience with something risqué.

Even the mildest suggestion of a threesome might be used to imply things about characters, like the dance lesson scene in *Dirty Dancing,* where Penny and Johnny sandwich Baby between them, as though that alone marks the two characters as not just older, but more worldly and experienced in very particular ways.

At the risk of dating myself, I saw the movie *Threesome* at a very impressionable age. If you're not familiar with it, the movie is about three college students (Lara Flynn Boyle, among others) who are accidentally roomed together on a college campus. The scandalous part? It's two men and one woman. And with the title, you know where this is going. I'm not saying it's a good movie, but it left a mark. The dynamics between the characters, the idea of multiple bodies, and the slight edge of homoeroticism all mesmerized me in those pre-internet days when smut was difficult to get ahold of, and before I knew there were communities of people into the same things as me.

Later, during my senior year of high school, *Wild Things* came out, and people were equal parts intrigued and scandalized. Once again, the threesome was shown as a way to brand the characters as brazen, or outside of society's norms.

Want to consume some threesome media of your own? Here's a nonexclusive list of options. These films or tv shows feature a threesome, group sex, or multi-person relationship or sexual dynamics:

Threesome (1994)
Wild Things (1998)
Shortbus (2006)
Y Tu Mamá También (2001)
Professor Marston and the Wonder Women (2017)
True Blood (series)
The Magicians (series)
Sirens (1994)
Sense8 (series)
Easy (series)
House of Cards (series)
Shame (2011)
Savages (2012)
Henry & June (1990)
Kinsey (2004)
American Psycho (2000)
Sex in the City (series)
Vicky Cristina Barcelona (2008)
The Dreamers (2003)

Try having yourself a little viewing party—not just to decide what feels hot to you, but to see if you can pick out any best practices, or any situations to avoid.

Threesomes in Porn

Porn can be a great way to get turned on or explore new kinks or new fantasies. But it's important to remember that's what porn is—a fantasy. Porn isn't sex ed or a how-to. And when it comes to threesome porn, it's often even more unrealistic than porn involving just two people.

Remember that porn is usually shot with a particular viewer in mind, and is often portraying a particular fantasy. As such, often one participant is the center of attention the whole time. While that can be hot for an outside viewer, it doesn't always work so well for a threesome you might try to have yourself.

Remember that in porn you're not seeing their negotiations or their check-ins. There's no acknowledgment of preexisting relationships. And you're missing any potential awkwardnessaboutchoosingpositions,orswitchingfromoneposeto another.

So use porn to get turned on or to come up with some fantasy ideas, but don't expect your real life threesome to look just like what you've seen on screen.

Historical Threesomes

Threesomes are far from a new idea, and I think it's safe to assume we've been having group sex for as long as we've been having any sex at all. (Even animals have been observed having threesomes![1])

Books and art from across cultures support our long-held fascination with threesomes. Perhaps the most well-known manual for sexual positions, *The Kama Sutra* contains multiple entries for threesomes. Images of threesomes also adorned the walls in the baths of Pompeii, and temples in India are decorated with carvings depicting group sex.

Moving closer to modern times, one of my favorite examples of group sex in art is The Cursed Woman (*La Femme Damnée*) by Octave Tassaert, painted in 1859. Despite what the title would have you believe, the woman in question seems to be having a lovely time.

WHY ARE PEOPLE INTO MULTIPERSON PLAY?

Let Me Count the Ways

Referring back to Lehmiller's book *Tell Me What You Want*, he states that group sex is the "single most popular sexual fantasy among Americans today," with a third of survey participants describing it as their favorite fantasy of all time.[ii]

Impressive, right? And that certainly aligns with the number of questions I hear on the topic. So if you're curious about threesomes, you're far from alone.

But why? Of all the things people can and do fantasize about, what is it about multiple bodies that makes this the top of the list? The following pages will explore some of the more common reasons people turn to this fantasy, and I bet you can come up with even more reasons of your own.

Lots of Stimulation

One of the key reasons people are excited by the idea of threesomes or multiperson sex is that they can involve a high level of stimulation. And that stimulation can come in many forms.

For starters, there are a lot of visual stimuli when there are extra people. Not only are there more lovely bodies to look at, but you're able to watch people doing things to each other in front of you, a perspective you simply don't get from one- or two-person sex.

There may be high levels of physical stimulation, too, especially if you spend time as the center of attention. More people can mean more hands, mouths, and genitals making contact with you, and that can be very exciting.

There can also be higher levels of auditory stimulation. Maybe there's dirty talk, maybe there are moans and gasps. All of this can be arousing to listen to.

Additional people can also mean new dynamics and fantasies to explore, which can help keep even the most active brain busy. Sometimes an extra pair of hands is incredibly useful, not to mention an extra mouth, when it comes to exploring these new fantasies.

On a basic level, desire for a threesome can harken back to some of our earliest sexual fantasies. Maybe even before we're fantasizing about particular people, we're fantasizing about body parts we'd like to play with and explore. That's a lot of stimulation! And a threesome can be a way to embody that early fantasy of many body parts at our disposal.

Voyeurism and Exhibitionism

Exhibitionists like being watched, and voyeurs like watching—what a perfect match! And while your mind might be jumping to flashers and Peeping Toms, both voyeurism and exhibitionism can be engaged in with the consent of all parties.

If you enjoy having an audience, having an extra person in the bedroom can be particularly exciting. Especially if they're someone new to you, it can be a big thrill to put on a show. While compliments and affirmations from our sweeties are wonderful, it can be extra stimulating to get that kind of attention from a new source. While I don't doubt the sincerity of long-term partners when they say nice things, I have heard from clients that they worry their partners, "have to say that." Whatever the reason, attention from a new source can be a big turn-on. And in the context of a threesome, you can share that extra arousal all around.

If you get a thrill out of visual stimuli, you can't beat a sex show happening right in front of you. It's hard to describe the sensual overload of bodies entangled in the bed with you. It's so rare in our culture to see other people having sex, that seeing it right in front of you can be an almost overwhelming amount to process (in a good way).

If you're having a threesome with a regular partner, it can be incredibly fulfilling to watch other people appreciate how beautiful or skilled they are. It can actually inflate our own ego to see a partner of ours receiving compliments, while at the same time we can appreciate them getting that feedback from a new source. I absolutely love hearing a partner of mine receive compliments. Another bonus you can get from an additional partner as an audience is the ability to share your partner's vulnerability with another person. There's something incredibly tender that can happen during sex, and allowing someone else into that space can feel very special.

There's also a particular pleasure in taking pride in your partner getting someone else off. Like being in the stands while your favorite team scores a goal, you can cheer on your partner as they execute especially sexy moves.

Personally, I enjoy both voyeurism and exhibitionism, and that make threesomes an ideal scenario. In fact, I enjoy watching so much that I sometimes have to remind myself to participate! More than once I've caught myself at the foot of the bed, enjoying watching the people in front of me, only to remember that I should dive in and help out. The same is true at sex parties—I'm often found curled up on the couch simply enjoying the scene in front of me. And that's a totally valid way to participate if it sounds like your jam. An extra person on hand to pass over a sex toy or extra lube is always appreciated.

There's even evidence that voyeurism and third party play (or even just watching porn of it) can increase desire and virility.[iii] Whether or not this can consciously affect someone's desire for a threesome, there's clearly some deep-seated psychology at play when we're rolling around with more than one other person.

Here's what one woman had to say:

> My partner and I had been wanting to invite this person to join us for years! My partner knew them years before they met me, and I was introduced to them through our common queer circle. They are a performer, and my partner and I would often go to their performances just to adore them from afar. One fateful night at our local sex club queer night, we ran into them and they weren't working the party for once! We invited them into a private room, had the safer-sex talk, and fucked until the venue closed for the night! It was my first time being able to watch my partner fuck someone else, and it was truly one of the hottest moments I've experienced.
>
> I am both a voyeur and an exhibitionist, so threesomes and group sex are very attractive to me. This experience solidified further what I already knew: the more, the merrier!

Cuckolding

One common fantasy that involves the addition of a third person is that of cuckolding. Classically, this involves a man and a woman, with the man watching his partner with another man.

While this can fall under the banner of nonmonogamy in general or threesomes in particular, there are some specific ways this fantasy plays out.

The *cuckold* in this situation is the man who is watching his partner with someone else. The term has been around in several variations since the Middle Ages, originally referring to a man who was being cheated on. These days, however, the term primarily refers to the consensual fetish.[2]

One of the most common ways to indulge in this fantasy is for the cuckold to be in the room, perhaps in a chair with a good view of the bed, while he watches his partner with another man. Of course, the genders can be mixed up in any way you'd like. For a complete gender reversal, the term cuckqueen is sometimes used.

While the partner on the outside of the experience is most usually in the room to watch, the fantasy can also be indulged in from afar, by receiving pictures or even simply hearing stories of the adventures they missed out on.

Consensual cuckolding can be hot for any number of reasons, many of which align with the pleasures of voyeurism or exhibitionism. But there can be an added element in the mix, of feeling jealousy and being able to channel that into an erotic charge.

This jealousy can play out with a hot "reclaiming" scene once the third has left, which allows the existing couple to enjoy all of that erotic build-up between themselves.

Taking cuckolding to a kink or BDSM context, there is sometimes an element of humiliation involved in cuckolding as a fetish, though that's certainly not required. This can be part of

---

2   An unsettling element of how this fetish sometimes plays out is wanting the third man to be black—bringing racial and racist elements into play. To align with the philosophy of this book, cuckolding should be engaged in only with the full enthusiastic consent of everyone involved, and while treating everyone with the utmost respect. Read more about race and partner choice in Chapter 21.

a wider power dynamic within the relationship, or something reserved for these specific encounters. On the other side, there can be elements of power play for the partner who is taking a new lover in view of their existing partner. When this is the element being played up, you'll sometimes hear the term, *Hotwife*. In this instance, it's the "wife" or female partner whose behavior is being discussed or centered, whereas "cuckold" refers to the husband or man in the situation.

Like most kink play, there are countless ways this can play out, and numerous ways to balance the power exchange—if that's an element you'd like to include.

Here's how one man describes a scenario that can fall into the cuckolding category:

About a decade ago I was hanging out with some friends of mine, a married couple, whom I hadn't seen for some time. We'd made a night of it going from bar to bar, and toward what I thought was the end of the evening we had a pause in the conversation. The couple looked at each other and then the wife looked at me.

"Have you ever been propositioned by your friend's wife?" she said.

I was surprised. I was also immediately aroused, as I'd always found her very attractive. I said no and looked to my other friend, who had a big grin on his face. I asked him if he was okay with this. He said, "I love it. It's like my own private porno starring my wife."

It's not a humiliation thing. Rather, he loves sharing her with guys he trusts. She loves getting fucked and having attention lavished upon her.

We have met up consistently since then, for over a decade now. It's actually my longest-lived sexual relationship, and

I hook up with them every six months or so. He likes to call her a naughty girl. And she likes to be one.

It's also worth noting that being in a threesome with a guy who is not into other dudes still requires trust and intimacy, and even sexual intimacy of a sort. He's never once made any homophobic jokes or comments about me, my sexuality, or how we pretty consistently get naked and vulnerable together. It's instructive and positive to express masculinity with other guys in such a nontoxic manner, and to have a mutual partner be a form of camaraderie rather than jealousy or rivalry.

Also, it's nice to know you can tag in a friend for an assist when you're fucking someone insatiable.

Exploration of New Bodies and New Dynamics

Every body is different. They look different, smell different, taste different, and are capable of different things. A position that might be terrible for one person's knees might be someone else's favorite. A particular act that someone loves won't be everyone's cup of tea. By adding new people to the mix, you've got a chance to explore all kinds of new things.

This is one of the benefits of relationships with some degree of openness. They let you have experiences with people you might not have if you're only dating (or having sex) to find a nesting partner. There are people who could be a bad fit for you to make a life with, but who still have a lot to offer.

Threesomes can work that way, too. You're exploring with people you might not want to pair up with for the long term, but who are still wonderful in many ways.

You're also getting to see and experience new combinations of bodies—as well as contrasts between bodies. With a three-some, you're not only exploring new people yourself, there are three of you exploring. And that means you're seeing people combine in new and novel ways. Kissing a woman's soft lips and then immediately kissing a man's bearded face. Stroking someone's soft body and curves and then feeling someone's taught muscles.

Sometimes we're better able to notice and appreciate things about people when they're highlighted by contrasts. And threesomes allow you to notice many beautiful contrasts between people.

Specific Fantasies

Do you have a fantasy that simply requires an extra person? The thing about threesomes is that they can help facilitate many of the most common fantasies that people have.

Interested in BDSM but your partner isn't? Bring in a third. Interested in exploring with someone of a different gender? Add them to the mix. Think the idea of sex with a stranger is hot? You guessed it, invite one home.

Not only does a new or extra person help realize many common fantasies, but doing it in the context of a threesome provides some structure, stability, and safety if you're bringing along a friend or partner.

Here are some fantasies you might try to fulfill:

- Kissing someone new while your partner watches.
- Trying out the fabled three-way kiss.
- Having multiple hands on your body at once.
- Feeling a mouth on each nipple at the same time.
- Experiencing multiple penetration.
- Sleeping in a three-way cuddle puddle.
- Watching your partner try new things.

Arousal Feedback Loop

Again and again, people come to my office and say that the biggest turn-on for them is when their partner is turned on. It can even become a problem, when two people are so focused on the other person that neither one is able to get that particular need met.

Bringing in extra people is a great way to watch your partner get turned on and experience pleasure. Who doesn't like the occasional helping hand?

With more stimulation and more combinations of bodies and sex acts there are a lot of opportunities for arousal and pleasure, and if seeing another person aroused or experiencing pleasure is a big turn-on . . . you see how this goes?

If seeing someone else's pleasure is a big turn-on for you, then why not double that pleasure with two people to watch? It can finally give you the outside perspective that can be missing from two-person sex. You'll be able to watch your partner get turned on and enjoy themselves either from a slight distance, or while you chip in yourself. The possibilities for these combinations are endless.

Taboo

Taboo can be a huge turn-on. It's also very culturally specific. In mainstream western culture, monogamy is the norm, so anything that breaks that norm can have the thrill of the taboo. For that reason alone, threesomes have great potential for taboo play.

If you're part of an existing couple, there's the excitement of breaking norms by seeing a partner flirt with, kiss, and even have sex with another person. And if you're the third, playing with the taboo of being an interloper—the "other man" or "other woman"—can be a hot fantasy to explore, even if it's kept as a personal thrill.

Threesomes have the opportunity to break a number of other taboos as well.

In western culture, people socialized as women are often shamed for wanting sex, let alone with two people at once. So any expression of desire can bring a bit of a charge to an encounter—especially if mixed with other taboo or wanton activities, like double penetration.

Some people lean into this taboo by adding role play or dirty talk, wanting to be "shamed" for these desires within the safe container of consensual play. If this sounds like you, consider negotiating some name-calling, like "slut" or any other words that feed into this particular fantasy for you.

In a threesome involving two straight or mostly straight men, there's a charge from pushing the boundaries of sexuality. Whether it's negotiated as being focused on the third, or whether the men explore a bit with each other, too, the added thrill of taboo is there. Cultural homophobia is a big elephant in the room, so whether you acknowledge it or not, it's likely to play some part in how you're feeling during this kind of group scenario. And that's another fantasy you can lean into if it strikes your fancy. Why not add some locker room role-play, or some other scenario that intentionally enhances this taboo?

Just remember that adding intentional taboo play to the mix is a significant leveling up, so make sure you're ready for the added emotional complexity.

Exploring Sexuality

There are a lot of reasons people might not have explored all of their attractions and turn-ons. From cultural or familial stigma to simple lack of opportunity, we can get pretty far along in life and realize there are things we're still curious about.

Trying new things can be scary, and that's one of the reasons that interests can go unexplored. For some, it can feel safer to explore something new with the support of an existing partner or friend in the room. That's why threesomes can be a great way to try new activities—you can have the added safety and comfort of a trusted person right there with you.

Any time you're exploring something new, it's important to be transparent with the other people involved. In the case of a threesome, make sure the new person or people know where you're coming from, or if you're uncertain. While lots of people enjoy helping others explore and experiment, it won't be for everyone.

In a threesome to explore sexuality, it's especially important to have not just a plan A, but plans B, C, and even D. In the moment you might find that you're scared or uncomfortable, or even just not as turned on as you'd hoped, but still curious enough that you want to keep going.

Consider what activities you want to have on the table, and what feels like going too far. Maybe you want to stick to things like kissing with the new person, while you explore how that feels. Or maybe touching everywhere with hands feels comfortable, but you're not ready to explore oral sex on a new body.

Whatever lines feel most comfortable for you are fine, as long as you communicate them to the other person in advance and they feel good about it. And remember that it's probably better to start small and see how it goes than to try to squeeze everything in to one adventure. If things go well and you want more, you can always make another date with the same person, or line up another threesome partner. But if you move past your own comfort zones, you can't take that back later.

Another reason a threesome can be a good method of exploration is that you've got a pinch hitter in the room. So, if you realize you've gone as far as you're ready to go with a new person, there are a wide variety of things that can still happen. Maybe the other person takes the lead and you can just watch. More people means more possibilities, and that can make it feel safer to dive in.

Simple Curiosity

With so many cultural references to threesomes, it would be hard not to have some curiosity. Just what is all the fuss about? Curiosity is a wonderful motivation for any kind of exploration.

Whether it's curiosity about the dynamic of three bodies in a bed, of watching sex in front of you, or of exploring with someone new, we all crave novelty and new experiences.

Why Do YOU Want a Threesome?

As with any kind of sex, knowing *why* you want to do it is as valuable as knowing *what* you want to do.

Have you ever thought about why you want sex at any given time? One study found 237 reasons![iv] Think about it: if you want sex because you're looking for touch and connection, and the other person is just looking for an orgasm (both valid reasons!), the sex is going to look different for each of you. So it's important to know the why in order to help determine the how.

What does this have to do with threesomes? Well, the "why" of your threesome will help determine a lot of the details you need to decide on. If part of the why is exploring with someone of a particular gender, then that determines the gender of the additional person you're looking for. If the why is to explore a particular BDSM dynamic, then the person you're looking for needs to be into and experienced with that dynamic.

If you're planning a threesome with a friend or partner, it's also important to make sure your reasons for wanting a threesome are in alignment. For example, if you're excited about exploring with another man, but your partner doesn't want another man in the room—there's an issue to address. Or if one of you wants a wild night never to be spoken of again, and the other is curious about a triad relationship—again, there had better be a conversation.

Even for more subtle differences in your *whys*, it's worth having the conversation with your friend or partner to make sure there's enough overlap in what you're looking for to move forward. And whether you're solo or partnered, it's a good idea to have the *why* conversation with your potential threesome playmates, too, to make sure everyone's reasons align.

Challenging Cultural Assumptions

Our culture is constantly policing what's acceptable. From acceptable gender presentation to acceptable relationship styles, people outside the norm hear about it. And while this is beginning to shift, we've all grown up steeped in these cultural "norms."

If you've always been monogamous, or surrounded by monogamous couples—not to mention a primarily monogamous culture—you're likely to have some monogamy baggage. And if you're thinking of opening a monogamous relationship—even if only for the occasional threesome—you're going to feel cultural pushback, even if it's all internal.

Mainstream monogamy culture tells us that one person is meant to fill all of our needs forever. Not only that, but being monogamous is supposed to mean that you never find anyone else attractive.

Neither of these things is true, or even possible, and if we try to hold our partner to these standards, we're forcing them to lie to us. Still, it can be a big jump to go from saying a particular actor in your favorite show is cute, to swiping Tinder for a threesome buddy. And it's natural for this to bring up feelings.

You're going to have to spend some time exploring those feelings to see where they're coming from. It can take some time to figure out if the root of an emotion is a value that you hold, or a value the mainstream culture holds.

What other cultural baggage might you need to release? Maybe the idea that being attracted to someone you're not partnered to means there's something wrong with your relationship. Or that jealousy is both inevitable and a sign of how much you care.

See if you can think about all of the assumptions you have about relationships in general, and about your relationship in particular, and then see if those assumptions are serving you. You get to choose what kind of relationship you want to have—you don't need to bend to cultural prescriptions.

ARE THREESOMES FOR YOU?

Check In with Yourself

Whether you're solo or partnered, the first step before trying something new is to check in with yourself. Where is the idea of having a threesome coming from? Is it something you've fantasized about for yourself, or something a partner brought up?

While it can be very tempting to go along with things our partners are excited about, it's important to take a time out and check in with ourselves first, outside the influence of someone else's desires. Do you meditate? Journal? Go for long walks? Whatever style of self-reflection works for you is what you should employ here.

Spend some time rolling the idea of a threesome around in your mind. What comes up for you? Is there a list of things that sound hot that you're excited to try? Or do you feel yourself getting anxious about things that could go wrong, or that might feel tricky or awkward in the moment?

Take some time to actually write these reactions down. Grab a journal and pour your thoughts out until there's nothing left.

First, make a list of all the things you're excited to do with a threesome.

Next, make a list of all your fears. Be honest with yourself and get them down on the pages.

Do this self-reflection process long enough to give every thought and feeling a chance to bubble to the surface, and then see if the pros outweigh the cons. If you decide to move forward with a threesome, use the sections in this book to work through the areas that feel scary to you so that you can get to an enthusiastic yes before diving in.

Quiz/Checklist

Here are some questions for you to consider:

- ▶ What are you hoping to get from a threesome experience?
- ▶ What are the most common elements of your sexual fantasies?
- ▶ How do you feel when someone else mentions a threesome (or it comes up in media)?
- ▶ Do you like to share?
- ▶ Do you feel comfortable having sexually explicit conversations?
- ▶ Does it turn you on to see other people turned on?
- ▶ Are you comfortable being seen naked from various angles?
- ▶ If you have an existing partner, do you like seeing them with other people?
- ▶ Do you feel comfortable negotiating for what you want and need?
- ▶ Do you feel comfortable setting boundaries?

▸ If you have a partner, do you trust them to respect your boundaries?

▸ Are you ready to say no, even if it might disappoint other people?

▸ Do you feel able to have conversations about sexual health and safety?

▸ Why do you want a threesome?

▸ Does this reason align with the people you're going to play with?

▸ What is your risk tolerance when it comes to sexual safety?

▸ What is your risk tolerance when it comes to emotional safety?

▸ What have your best sexual experiences involved?

▸ Do you think threesomes can be a safe and healthy form of sexual exploration?

▸ Do you feel confident in your own sexiness?

How Do You Feel Your Feelings?

How in touch with your feelings are you? When you're having a strong emotion or a sudden reaction, can you name it? Can you describe what you're feeling to other people? And do you have ways to soothe yourself?

If you're going to engage in threesomes (or really, any sex at all) you're going to need to speak up about your feelings.

Have you ever thought about where your feelings live in your body? In a physical sense, where do you feel different feelings? If you don't already know, it can be helpful to start paying attention. Maybe take notes or keep a journal while you're learning how your emotions and your body align.

While this is simply a useful life skill, it's relevant for threesomes because your body often knows how you're feeling before your mind does. And the sooner you can feel an issue coming on, the sooner you can address it.

What does anxiety feel like in your body? How is that different from excitement?

For me, bad anxiety is a flutter in my chest, and anticipation or excitement is a little lower, in my belly. The feelings are pretty similar, and I need to pay attention to know which is which.

I use this trick on myself all the time. I used to do theater and got very used to the feeling of what I was calling stage fright before every show. But true stage fright can be paralyzing. That wasn't what I was experiencing. For me, that nervous energy translated into exactly the kind of energy I needed on stage to give a good performance.

A mentor helped me realize this was exactly what I was feeling before I went to teach classes. I thought I was anxious about every class. But really, it was that same nervous excitement about getting on stage. And coming to that realization has changed my relationship to teaching.

When our body is feeling something, our mind looks for a way to justify it. So if it feels what might be nerves, it comes up with lists of things you could be nervous about. And the next thing you know, you're worried about everything from when you need to change your oil to filing your taxes.

This same impulse can work in our favor, too. It's why smiling can actually put you in a better mood. Or standing in the superhero pose can make you more confident. Our mind believes what our body is doing.

Use all of this to your advantage.

Track where the bad kind of nerves and anxiety live in your body. Then you'll start to feel the warning signs. And you'll be able to get some advance warning when you're getting into a situation you don't feel good about—which means you can change course or stop it sooner.

It also means that if you want to psych yourself up, you can smile and take confident poses. Fake it until you feel it, basically. But only if that's in line with what you really, deeply want.

So learn to check in with yourself because I'm going to keep suggesting that throughout this book. Get used to giving your body a mental scan, looking for where feelings are living, and giving them a name.

5

BABY STEPS TO EXPLORE THREESOMES

Exploration

It's hard to predict how you'll feel having your first threesome, even if it's something you've fantasized about. There are a lot of emotional aspects to consider, along with the logistics, especially if you're part of an established couple.

If you're not sure how you'll feel seeing your partner turned on by another person, there are some ways you can slowly explore before inviting another person into your bedroom.

Work through the suggestions in this section, and then back up and try the exercises at the end of the previous chapter to check in with yourself again. Does anything change?

Nonsexual Nudity

Backing up a big step—it's worth considering how our culture handles bodies, even when it's not about sex. In some countries, nude beaches, spas, and baths are the norm. And people grow up seeing a variety bodies hanging out nude. If you grew up in the US, and weren't part of one of those cultures, casual nudity probably wasn't your experience.

Before getting ready to see other people naked in a sexy context, it can help to build a general comfort around bodies. Depending where you live, you may have access to nude beaches, or nude spa or soak venues. These spaces are entirely nonsexual—and that's the point—making them a great start.

For those of us who grew up without access to nonsexual nudity, it can be valuable to experience a range of bodies beyond what we usually see in the media. It can also be a careful first step to simply see how you, or you and a partner, feel around other naked bodies.

At the very beginning of my first year in college, I was invited to a spa in Santa Cruz. It was described to me as a beautiful outdoor space with multiple soaking tubs, both cold and hot, as well as a sauna. This sounded like a dream, and I agreed right away. It was only hours later that it was brought to my attention that this was a nude space. Co-ed naked hot tubbing. As an 18-year-old from Los Angeles, I was not prepared.

I told myself that college meant new experiences, and so I should give it a try. I then spent the rest of the time I had to get ready standing in front of my dorm room mirror, trying to decide which hairstyle went best with naked.

Joking aside, this was a big deal for me. Like most teenagers, I was far from comfortable with my body. And while I'd had one sex partner, and had seen people dressing and undressing backstage of theater productions, I'd never simply seen people hanging around naked.

Luckily we were there after dark, and were largely under the water. But even so, it was an eye-opening experience. I got to see more than twenty people—of all genders and body types—simply enjoying themselves and their bodies, in an entirely nonsexual context.

That spa, and the other one like it in town, became regular features of my college experience, and helped form how I view bodies today.

★ ★ ★

If you decide to give this a try, keep proper etiquette in mind. If you're going to a spa or soaking venue, read everything on the website before you go. There are likely specific rules to follow; everything from bringing your own towel or shower sandals, to rules against wearing sunglasses. I ran into the sunglasses rule at a Portland spa—apparently it creeps people out because they can't tell if they're being looked at. That never would have occurred to me, but it's a good point!

If you're going somewhere like a nude beach, there likely won't be a website with specific guidelines or rules. So follow your best common sense. Remember that these spaces are nonsexual and there may be children present. That means no engaging in sexual activity and no lewd behavior. Don't stare and don't hit on people.

Instead, bask in the rare joy of sun and sand on your skin. Think about how many sensual experiences we can have that aren't about sex, and yes—enjoy the presence of other people without a sexual context.

Both while you're in the space and after, check in with yourself about how you're feeling. Are issues of shame or fear or comparison coming up for you? If so, you may want to do some work around that before diving deeper.

Doing self work can be an uncomfortable process, but the results are well worth it. One of the easiest ways to begin this process is by journaling. The process of writing out your thoughts and feelings can help you discover more about what's going on, as well as possibly some of the root causes of the emotions.

If you find yourself having overwhelming reactions, that could be a sign that working with a therapist or coach could be helpful. Delving into sexual exploration can unearth emotional landmines, and professional help can be a valuable resource.

Strip Clubs

When you're ready to explore a sexual environment, consider giving strip clubs a try. If you've never been to a strip club before, the idea can be intimidating, but with a little research you can go in feeling prepared.

There are a wide range of strip clubs available depending on where you live. Large cities have more options than smaller ones, and laws vary state by state. For example, some states allow full nudity in places with alcohol (like Oregon, where I live) and some don't (like Washington and California). There are other state laws that influence what the shows are like and how close dancers can get to visitors, so keep this section in mind for general advice, but check out the websites and reviews of clubs near you for more specific information.

While strip clubs featuring female dancers are more common, there are plenty of clubs with male dancers, as well as clubs that feature trans or queer strip nights—especially in larger cities. So be sure to do a little research before deciding whether clubs are for you—there may be a lot more options than you've realized.

A strip club adventure is not necessarily cheap. Some clubs have a door fee, and you'll need cash on hand for tipping. A general guideline is to tip at least a dollar per song when you're watching someone dance, but of course more is appreciated. If you're going to get a private dance, that's another expense. Generally private dances/lap dances start at around twenty dollars per song, but this varies by region and club. Some clubs also offer VIP rooms or champagne rooms, and the prices of those spaces will vary.

Remember that like any adventure we discuss in this book, it's always okay to change your mind and leave. Maybe you're only in the club for a few minutes before you decide it's not for you—that's okay. It's still a valuable learning experience.

The vibe from strip club to strip club is variable, so just

because you don't like one club doesn't mean all strip clubs aren't your jam. Again, see what you can figure out from online reviews before you go, so you have the best chance of finding one that's to your taste.

Why go to a strip club? Unlike at nude beaches, at a strip club it's okay to stare. (Make sure you're tipping anyone you're watching!) It's also okay to be aroused. So, while seeing nonsexual nudity can give you a lot of valuable information about yourself, there's a whole new set of information you can learn here.

When you're settling in to a club, choose your position and your view. Most strip clubs will have a *rack*, or bar, around the stage where you can sit for a closer look, while also having tables around the room and perhaps a standard bar to sit at as well. Depending on the club, the dancers may be the main feature, or may be a sideline to a bar or even something like video poker.

If you're entering a club for the first time, hang back for a bit to get your bearings. Maybe sit at a table where you can watch the whole room and get a sense of the place and how other patrons are behaving. The vibe in a club can be anything from super sleepy, with one or two regulars hanging around, to incredibly rowdy, with a bachelor party or two raging along.

If you're feeling okay after you've settled in, try for a seat close to the stage. Some dancers will interact with customers a bit, and this can be a great way to test out sharing that kind of attention.

If you came with a partner, how does it feel to watch your partner watching someone else? Is it sexy to see them interested in or excited by another person? Be honest with yourself and acknowledge any reactions that come up.

While many strip clubs have bars, stay sober enough to stay in touch with your feelings.

If watching stage dances feels sexy and fun, try a private dance together. That way you'll get to see your partner up close and personal with another person, which gives you another chance to test how you'll feel in a threesome.

Depending on the club, a private dance could happen behind a closed door, behind a curtain, or simply in an out of the way corner. But the rules are the same—don't touch the dancers! The easiest way to remember this can be to sit on your hands.

In some cases, a dancer may invite some touching—but wait to be asked, and don't make any assumptions. It's a great idea to talk all of this through with your partner before going to a club so you don't have to make any snap decisions in the moment. Are private dances even on the table if you're both feeling good at the club? If so, is touching an option if you're invited?

Even if you're not touching the dancers (and you probably aren't) they'll be touching you. While the amount of touch varies, it's called a lap dance for a reason, and the dancer will be up close and personal.

Does it feel hot to see someone else touching your partner? To see them turned on? If this is a brand new experience for the two of you, you're likely to feel a little overwhelmed with new reactions and new information. Give yourself a couple days to process and see what comes up.

What about talking about the experience afterwards? Do you enjoy sharing tales from your strip club date night? Is it hot to talk about which dancers you each liked the most? Or to fantasize about what happened, or what could have happened?

Sometimes an adventure like this can really kick-start conversations and dirty talk because you'll have some basis for understanding what interacting with a third person really feels like.

And yes, those dancers are people too! While strip clubs are an easier test run because of the defined boundaries, dancers need to be treated with respect. You're going to their place of work, and their time is valuable. Make sure you're tipping for any and all interactions, even when you're simply watching from the sidelines.

And if you do have tricky feelings come up in the moment, take the conversation outside, or at least away from the stage. Don't let the dancers get caught in any relationship conversation crossfire.

What about if you're flying solo? You can still try this route for exploration! Even on your own, a strip club can be a great way to see how you feel in a shared, sexually charged environment. And at many clubs you can get a private dance from two dancers at once, which is a great option for seeing how you feel about having three people in a room.

Do you enjoy watching two people up close, or do you find that you want the attention on yourself? Is watching people touch each other (or even kiss each other) right in front of you a fantasy come true, or does it feel awkward? How you respond to a situation like this certainly isn't a perfect indicator for how a threesome would feel, but it can give you some important clues to your reactions to help you know which directions to aim your future exploration.

Sex Parties

If sex clubs or play parties are available in your city (they probably are!), they can be another great way to explore and figure out your comfort zone. We'll talk about going to sex parties to meet threesome partners later on, but for now, let's discuss parties for the voyeuristic and exploratory aspect.

Before going out, be sure to read all the rules of the party or club you plan to attend. Every space has its own culture, and the more you know before heading out, the more comfortable you'll be. As you're checking out websites or event listings, keep an eye out for the following:

A tour of the space—many venue websites will have virtual tours or at least interior photos of the club so you can get a sense of what you'll be walking in to. Some clubs have many different spaces and private rooms, and some are one big open space—loft style. Each physical layout will lead to a different vibe and different party environment, so think about what will be the best fit for you.

Many clubs also have bars and dance floors. Even if you're not a drinker or a dancer, this means that there will be space set aside for socializing, which can be helpful for easing into the space.

Regardless of the layout, there will almost always be some buffer between where you walk in and where play actually happens.

Dress code—some spaces try hard to maintain an upscale environment and may not allow guests to wear jeans, shorts, sneakers, or other casual garb. In general, you don't need to look over the top sexy. Something you'd wear on a first date or to the theater usually works well. Slacks and a button up shirt or a little black dress, for example.

Lockers and showers—if you're going to bring items you don't want to carry around with you, from purses to sex toys, it's helpful to know if there's a locker room. Many clubs offer this option, but you may need to bring your own lock. Also, when there are showers available there are usually towels, too, but keep an eye out for details on the website.

Some clubs even have hot tubs or saunas. If you think that's something you might enjoy, but aren't ready for nudity, bring along a swimsuit.

Safer sex supplies—what supplies does the club provide? It can give you a sense of the space to know what they consider essential, even if you're not planning to play on this visit. And it's always a good idea to keep your favorite supplies on hand anyway.

Membership and pricing—many sex clubs are membership based. This is often to comply with local or regional laws around public sex. Check the website to see if membership is required, and also what the door fees are. There are likely to be some nights of the week that are less expensive or that are geared towards newcomers. There may also be a newcomer night where membership is waived, or a trial membership option.

So what about when you've read all the rules, gotten dressed up, and gone to the club? For the purposes of exploration, this sex club field trip is just about watching. Again, double-check the party rules, but at most spaces it's perfectly acceptable to simply watch. After all, voyeurism is participation.

You'll probably check in at some kind of front desk before you enter the space. You may be able to ask for a tour or ask any last questions you may still have.

Going to a sex party can work in a similar way to a strip club—but in addition to seeing other people in various states of undress, you may even see people having sex. How is that going to work? It depends on the space.

Many clubs will have some open areas where play is taking place. This can be anything from nude dancing, to making out, to explicit sex acts. Follow the cues of those around you for etiquette. Like in a strip club, this is a "look but don't touch" scenario. Allow some personal space between you and whomever you're watching, and refrain from any commentary—as tricky as that might be!

While you're doing all of this, be sure to keep checking in with yourself. It's okay to change your mind and head out at any time. How does it feel to be in a sexually charged environment? If you're with someone, how does it feel to share that space with a partner?

If everything is feeling good so far, this may also be an opportunity to try flirting with someone in this kind of an environment. Or, if you're with a partner, to watch your partner flirt with another person. Or maybe this is something you want to save for a second visit, once you're more comfortable with the space.

When you decide to give flirting a try, maybe one or both of you approach a single person or a couple and just start chatting. Or maybe you give each other a little space and watch from across the room to see what it feels like to view the interaction from a distance. There don't have to be any specific goals here. Just explore the interactions.

After your sex club adventure, take a few days to process your feelings. It can be helpful to journal, if that format works for you. If you went with a partner, give yourself a chance to compose your thoughts, and then talk together about the experience.

What emotions came up? What was the most exciting part? Did you get ideas for things you'd like to try? These conversations can be just as valuable, if not more so, than the club adventure itself.

Virtual Threesomes

You can also try a test run with a third party by exploring phone sex (it still exists!) or cam sites. For some folks, it can feel safer when the other person isn't in the same room, but you still have a chance to explore multiperson dynamics.

Like all the other exploration options discussed, be sure to negotiate your boundaries before you bring other people into the mix. If certain topics are off limits, make sure you explain that to whomever you'll be talking to.

If you'd like to try phone sex with a partner, simply use the speakerphone option. This can give you a chance to try a sexy scenario with another person, while at the same time maintaining a lot of distance, which may feel safer.

If you're more interested in a visual component, check out the numerous cam sites available. You can start by simply watching a public show with your partner—similar to watching at a strip club—and if you want to take it to the next level, you can pay for a private show.

In private, you'll be able to talk directly and make requests. Some sites even have an option for the cameras to work both ways, if you'd like the performer to watch you, too. This is a great option for finding out if you enjoy having an audience or showing off with your partner. Do you want to hear how sexy you look together? Do you want to see what flirting and sexy interactions look like, but with the safety of some extra distance? Cam sites might be a great option.

Cam sites each have their own pay structure. On some you can watch public shows (after creating a profile) without paying any money. On some you may be required to tip, or you may only be required to tip to join in on conversation. Regardless of the requirements, if you're watching the show, it's good form to tip.

If you'd like to move to the private show option, you'll have to pay for it. Again, each site will have their own way of handling it, but many of them have you pay by the minute. So not only is negotiating in advance a good idea for your relationship, it's a good idea to know what your requests are of the performer before you switch to a private room.

Just like with the strip club option, remember that phone sex operators and cam performers are people too—just because you're paying for time doesn't mean there are different standards for politeness and respect. Be kind to whoever you talk to, and grateful for the service they provide.

★ ★ ★

It's also possible to have a phone or virtual threesome with someone you know. I once got to be a phone-in unicorn. A messenger chat window popped up on my screen that read, "I'm about to get a blow job, do you want to listen?"

The message was from a casual acquaintance and one time play-partner. They show up in my messages every so often, either asking for or offering a dirty picture—but this was something new.

In the spirit of adventure, and because I was free that moment, I replied in the affirmative and moments later my phone was ringing.

I'd been working from home and was still sitting at my desk. Both my friend and his partner greeted me and then they got down to business. Most of the sounds were difficult to place and required some help from my imagination to build a scene. While the two were mostly silent, aside from some moaning and heavy breathing, they engaged in a little bit of dirty talk—and that dirty talk included me. My friend would ask, "Do you like having Stella hear what a good slut you are?" And a mumbled reply would follow.

The whole call lasted less than ten minutes, with them both thanking me at the end. And while it wasn't an overwhelming turn-on, I did get a voyeuristic thrill out of getting to listen in, and it was certainly a nice break from my workday.

EXPLORING WITHOUT OTHER PEOPLE

Threesomes as Fantasy

Maybe after reading all the considerations about threesomes with real people, you've decided this is something that should stay in fantasyland—that's okay!

Having an active fantasy life, whether alone or shared with a partner, is a great way to bring new elements into sex. Fantasies can be incredibly vivid and satisfying. Fantasies don't let you down—they can go exactly the way you want them to.

When was the last time you really got lost in a daydream? For many of us, this pastime ends when we aren't spending hours a day in a classroom. But letting your mind wander is a valuable skill. The brain needs time to process. This is part of why you always hear about people getting great ideas while taking a shower—that's often one of the only times we pause to focus on just one thing, without access to any screens or distractions.

Having a rich fantasy life is valuable for everyone, whether you're partnered or not. Thinking up different scenarios is one of the best ways to figure out what you might like to try in real life, or to simply learn more about your own turn-ons.

If you're inclined towards writing, you can even get your fantasies down on paper or on screen. The process of writing helps ideas flow in a different way, and you might find characters and situations coming to life that you hadn't considered before, or hadn't taken time to develop.

If you need a little fantasy fodder, turn to the internet for still images of threesomes. It doesn't matter if you're attracted to the people, or if the positions look comfortable. Just find one element in each picture that can inspire a fantasy of your own.

Maybe one includes a shower, and you enjoy a long, lazy fantasy about bodies sliding together covered in soap. Maybe there's a hot tub, and you imagine the warmth and the bubbles as you all relax and get comfortable with the idea of kissing. Whatever catches your eye, try to run with it and see where the ideas take you.

Dirty Talk

One of the easiest ways to try out a fantasy is by exploring through dirty talk. While having sex with a partner, you can talk about what you'd do if a third person were there.

Keep in mind that dirty talk can push emotional buttons too, and it's important to negotiate first—just as you would a situation with additional people.

You can negotiate dirty talk with a partner just like you'd negotiate actual play. (For a more in-depth discussion of negotiation best practices, see Chapter 14.) In fact, it's an important step. Just because something is being talked about rather than acted out, doesn't mean there aren't still boundaries to be aware of. So if you're going to indulge in threesome fantasy dirty talk with a partner, set some ground rules.

First of all, make it clear that just because you're dirty talking about a threesome doesn't mean you want to have one in real life. The talk isn't a slippery slope into a negotiation. Having this agreement is essential to being able to lose yourself to the fantasy without worrying that your partner may think you want to do these things for real. Many people use fantasy talk as a way to introduce negotiation for new adventures, so make it crystal clear that's not what's happening here.

Next, negotiate the parameters of the fantasy the same way you'd negotiate the real thing:

> ▶ Who is fair game for the fantasy? Are you talking about a fantasy third that's someone one or both of you know, or are you making up a stranger?

> ▶ If you're making up a stranger, what gender are they? What characteristics do they have? This is where you make sure nothing about the fantasy person pushes buttons of real-life insecurities.

> ▶ What activities will take place? Even when it's all talk, people still have boundaries, and not all activities might feel fun to talk about.

Dirty talk can be daunting for some, especially if coming up with sexy ideas doesn't feel natural. It's okay for one person to drive the story and for the other to simply agree to statements and ask questions. You can use theater improv rules and have your own dirty talk version of "Yes, and . . ."

Not familiar with that game? Here's how it works: one person makes a statement and the other person agrees and adds something. So one person could say, "It would be so hot to watch someone ride your face right now," and the other person could respond, "Yes, and I'd love to feel you hold their hips as they move against me."

The person who is more comfortable with dirty talk or has more ideas for the fantasy can drive the story, while the other agrees and adds details.

★ ★ ★

When it comes to talking through a fantasy, the planning phase is often just as much fun as the sex acts. This is true across fantasies, not just for threesomes. In the case of playing with a third, talk about how you'll find the person. Did you see their profile online? What about them attracted you? Something about their appearance? Something they said?

How does the flirting go once you start messaging? Do they compliment you and your partner—talk about how cute you look together? Remember this is all fantasy, so why not use this opportunity to reinforce good feelings about your relationship.

What happens when you meet up? What's the first thing you think when you see the other person? How do they greet you? Maybe they hug each of you in turn, and you're immediately turned on by the way they smell, or the brush of their hair against the side of your face. Maybe their hand lingers on your arm while they lean in to hug your partner, making sure you still feel included.

Once you all sit down for drinks, how does the conversation go? Is there more playful flirting? Maybe your fingers even brush against each other, or you're sitting close enough to feel the press of their knee against yours.

Do you start talking about what might happen if you go home together? The possibilities of what the three of you could do? What have they been fantasizing about doing in bed with a couple? What positions have they been dreaming of?

As you can see, the planning phase of a threesome has so much potential for dirty talk you might not even get as far as talking about sex before you've worked yourselves up so much you've stopped talking.

Real life can work that way too. While a threesome might be your goal, don't forget that the whole process can be fun, sexy, and an opportunity for deepening connection.

Erotica and Porn

If you need more fantasy fodder, try picking up some erotica anthologies that focus on threesomes. You can use the stories to fuel your own fantasies or simply read the stories to yourself or out loud to a partner.

Anthologies are a great place to start because, with a collection of authors, it's more likely that some of the stories will be to your taste. With an anthology, if something isn't doing it for you, you can just skip ahead a few pages to the next story.

When reading, simply losing yourself in the story is a wonderful option. If you want to do a bit of homework, too, you can also use the stories to help figure out your likes and dislikes.

In each story, what are the elements that really speak to you or turn you on? What parts simply aren't to your taste? Figuring those things out can help you build your own likes and dislikes list that you can use for future negotiations, for your own future fantasies, or for choosing future reading material.

You can also do this as an exercise with a partner to start getting ideas flowing. Each of you can read the same story and make notes about likes and dislikes, and then come together and share your thoughts. If you're using this as a way to plan for a real life threesome, don't just consider the sex the characters are having, pay attention to the logistical and emotional aspects too. How did the characters meet? Did they know each other already or meet for the threesome? How are they interacting when they're together?

All of these things can give you clues about what you might enjoy for yourself, and what aspects are making you nervous. For any aspects that are making you nervous, you might want to talk through them with your partner before diving in and having an experience.

★ ★ ★

If visual smut is your thing, there's no shortage of threesome porn available. Keep in mind that finding porn you like can be a little trickier than finding erotica, because there are more elements that have to be to your taste. When you're reading, you can fill in a lot of the details yourself. With visual porn, everything has to be just right. You need to like all of the performers, the setting they're in, and the dialogue if there is any.

But tricky doesn't mean impossible, so don't get discouraged. You can also use porn to get ideas even if it's not an absolute turn-on. What positions are people in? What acts are they engaged in? You can take notes about your likes and dislikes here, too.

The porn you're watching doesn't even need to feature threesomes. You can watch coupled or solo sex and insert yourself, or you and a partner, into the fantasy. What would you do if you were there with them? How would you add yourself to the activities? You can brainstorm ways to include an extra person into coupled sex, without anyone feeling left out.

Just remember that porn is fantasy fodder, not sex ed. The performers are professionals with specialized skills, so don't expect your body or your partners' bodies to be able to do every-thing you see in porn. They get time off camera to warm up and lube up, and take breaks as needed.

Sex Toys

Believe it or not, the wide variety of sex toys now available means you can do a pretty good job of simulating a threesome fantasy without another person in the room.

If you have a hard time with suspension of disbelief, and you're worried about the realism of the toys, consider adding a blindfold to the mix. A blindfold can spice up any kind of sex because it makes you focus on your other senses. And when you're engaging in some kind of role-play—like a simulated threesome—it can make the dirty talk and sensations even more believable.

There are a lot of ways you could do this, but we'll go over a few options to get you started.

First up, the advanced option: a fucking machine. Multiple companies make these kinds of toys, so you'll have to do some research to see which one is right for you. They're also on the high end of the price spectrum. If you've seen fucking machines in porn, you might be assuming they're only for providing penetration, but some options also come with Fleshlight-like attachments for providing something to penetrate as well. Combined with a blindfold, some dirty talk, and stimulation from both a partner and the machine, this experience can be surprisingly realistic.

For another option, consider sex dolls. And while the full head-to-toe dolls might be the first thing that comes to mind, there are also toys that are only part of a body, such as just a torso, or just a pelvis, etc. While at first that could sound off-putting, it's amazing what some good lighting plus arousal can do.

With these dolls arranged in the bed just so, with pillows and blankets around them, it's easy to imagine the rest of the body is simply covered up. Especially if you're playing by candlelight. Again, this can be used with a blindfold for extra help in the fantasy department, and talk can add to the experience.

Either the fucking machine or doll options can be used to recreate many of the threesome sex positions we'll explore a little later on.

What about using toys to facilitate some of the other possible threesome benefits?

One of the nice things about exploring with other people is being able to experience different kinds of bodies, for different experiences and sensations. But toys can facilitate this too.

Try realistic dildos in a variety of sizes, textures, and colors.

This can not only allow for variety but perhaps open up new activities. For example, you can get a small toy for experimenting with anal sex. They even make toys for adding a dildo to someone who already has a penis—both cock ring style and strap-on harnesses. This way, you can achieve double penetration with just one person, and still have your hands free for other activities.

You can also try Fleshlights or other masturbation sleeves in a variety of styles. These can provide different textures and different amounts of pressure so you can play with novelty and variety.

Another option is to combine multiple toys with your usual play to explore high-stimulation scenarios. Maybe someone adds a butt plug or other anal toy to penetrative or oral sex. Maybe there's a vibrator added to the mix. Maybe some nipple clamps. Anything you can do to light up multiple erogenous zones at once will raise the stimulation factor of the experience.

WHEN THERE'S
AN EXISTING COUPLE

What Is a Couple?

There are a lot of different ways people can come together for sexual play, and depending on the backgrounds and connections of the people involved, the threesome dynamics will feel different. So it's important to think about your relationships and dynamics and how they'll play out.

When I say *couple* in this book, it's usually in reference to a romantic pair. But for the sake of threesome dynamics, any time two of the people have some history together that changes things. So that can mean a pair of friends or acquaintances coming into the adventure together, versus someone coming in entirely solo.

When you're thinking about your ideal threesome dynamics, think about the different energy in the room when there are two people who have a longstanding relationship, or two people who have been lovers before, or three people who have just met up.

There's no better or worse here, but it's worth thinking about how each person's preexisting connection will influence the threesome.

Couple's Privilege

Speaking of couples, *couple's privilege* is a term you may not have heard before, but it's a concept worth considering if you're planning to date or play as a couple.

First, some notes on language. In polyamorous circles, you're likely to hear the term *couple's privilege* to describe the advantage an existing couple may have in regards to relationships with third parties. Whether explicitly hierarchal or not, an existing couple has history, which leads to a greater understanding of each other's needs, and often an impulse to protect the relationship from potential interference.

While protecting a relationship isn't a bad thing, it's important to make sure it's done mindfully, in a way that doesn't harm other people the couple may engage with—either individually or together.

It must be pointed out that using the term *privilege* is not without baggage. The privilege ascribed to couples is not systemic in the same way as something like white privilege. Rather, the term is being used in this context to discuss the power dynamics at play.

It's also worth being aware of these dynamics because if you're part of a couple seeking to engage with single people, couple's privilege might be something they're already sensitive to—whether that's because they've experienced bad behavior from other couples, or the simple fact that our culture is arranged to benefit people who are in pairs.

I've personally run into the frustrations of trying to plan a vacation for one, only to be inundated with advertising for romantic getaways and couples' packages. Our whole society is built around people pairing off, and while an ever growing number of people are rejecting that framework, it's still the society standard.

In the context of threesomes, here's how I'm using it: the

couple has a chance to negotiate in advance and come to their own agreements, and the third gets to opt in or out, based on those agreements. While this is still a consensual arrangement, there's a power imbalance worth acknowledging, if not all parties were around for all negotiations. Are the couple's needs being given more importance or priority than the third's? That's a problem.

The couple also has some built-in support after the threesome. Especially if the couple lives together, there's additional time for snuggles and check-ins that the third won't get.

While it can be extremely important to have boundaries and understandings in place with your partner before a threesome, be mindful of how these agreements affect your third. Boundaries should be for and about you and your partner, not a list of rules for the third to follow.

If you find yourself preparing to give a list of instructions, or dos and don'ts, it might be time to rethink your approach.

Here's what one polyamorous friend, Chelsea, had to say on the topic:

> What I want to address is couple's privilege on a smaller and more intimate level. Because you are right that most privileges have to do with sweeping societal dis/advantages. I think for the purposes of threesomes, you are referring not to how a couple is treated by the world at large, but how they use their pre-existing structure to determine how a third gets treated.
>
> My nesting partner/spouse and I have had a lot of talks about making sure that anyone else involved with either or both of us gets treated as a whole person. They are not a toy, not an afterthought, not a pet. I don't get to decide what they are "allowed" in my home or with my person.

Now, what I'm talking about is dating/relationships, not necessarily a guest star for occasional adventures. Maybe that changes it? But if so, they still get an equal yes and an equal no in all negotiations. None of this "WE have decided this is how it's gonna go, play by our rules or gtfo" nonsense. That is not treating them like an entire person with agency and needs and feelings.

That said, in protection of my relationship, if I felt like someone invited in had unsafe/unethical practices, I would definitely put my foot down (and be listened to), so I know I'm still benefiting from an emotional hierarchy in a lot of ways.

I'll admit, I do want to protect my family, my home. But I think part of that is . . . the family that we agreed to build is not a monogamous one. I have to protect that too. I have to protect that we have decided that this is important to us and that the ethical practice of it is crucial to who we are.

Starting the Conversation

One of the more common questions I hear is someone wondering how to tell their partner about a kink they have, or a fantasy they want to try. It can be scary to ask for what you want. Asking creates vulnerability and opens you up to rejection. It can also be scary to ask for new things if you're worried it will hurt your partners' feelings. Some people think that asking for something new will sound like they're dissatisfied with their current sex life or partner. My first book, *Tongue Tied*, goes into great detail about having these conversations, and more, but here's some threesome-specific advice.

When you want to start a conversation that might be sensitive, choose your timing well. Make sure no one is in a rush and everyone is well fed and well rested. Then, ask if they're up for hearing a fantasy.

When you're talking about what you'd like, try to incorporate why you'd like it. For example, "You're so sexy, I think it would be really hot to see someone else touching you," or "You know I've been interested in exploring with other women, I think I'd feel more comfortable if you were there."

Including a feeling or a reason for your interest can help provide context and can help guide the conversation. It can also help pique the other person's interest, if the activity doesn't otherwise sound like their jam.

Think about the difference between, "Do you want to have a threesome?" and "I'm excited about the idea of a threesome, would you be willing to try that with me?" In the second example, there's vulnerability in sharing a desire, which is often met with more kindness than a simple fantasy stated out of the blue.

If you've been together for a while, and strictly monogamous, there's more than one conversation between you and a threesome. It's a good idea to take a while and think the idea through, and process any feelings that come up, before diving in with another person.

If this conversation comes up out of the blue, the other person is likely going to be a bit shocked, and they might take some time to process their feelings. Many of us don't do well when put on the spot. Consider bringing up the topic while at the same time saying you're not expecting to make a decision right away, or anytime soon. Maybe something like, "I'd love to tell you about a fantasy I have, would that be okay?" And then if they're on board, "I've been thinking it would be really hot to have a threesome with you. I also know it's a big step and I'm not in any rush to come to a decision. Would you be up for thinking about it? Maybe we can just start by talking about it as a fantasy and see if it's a turn-on for us?"

When you offer to give someone time to think—or someone

asks for time—make sure you actually give it to them! All too often someone is excited to do or try something new, and they begin to nag about it. This is often when people land in my office. The subject of the new thing has become a sore spot because a partner keeps pushing. Sometimes it can help to agree to table the discussion for a set period of time. Maybe six months. And then revisit and see how everyone is feeling.

Remember that *how* you ask can be as important as what you're asking for. If you ask in a way that makes someone feel bad, or you keep pushing before they're ready to talk, you might sour them on the idea even if they might otherwise have been up for it.

Try to keep your excitement in check and remember that everyone comes around to new things at their own pace. You're better off starting slow and having the chance to move forward together, rather than souring them on the idea and making it a no-go forever.

How Much Time Are You Dedicating?

Are threesomes a fun fantasy that you might get around to at some point, or are they something you're determined to make happen as soon as possible? It's helpful to get on the same page about what priority this fantasy takes and how much time you're willing to dedicate to it.

Like anything to do with sex and relationships, it's important that it doesn't become a chore. If you're finding that threesome planning is taking up all of your time together, that could mean it's time to take a break.

Threesomes are going to be the best when the relationship is in a strong place, so maintaining your intimacy and connection during this process is vital. Make sure you're still going on dates and having fun, hot sex on your own so that adding someone feels like an adventure, not like a requirement.

In fact, this is a great time to level up the sex you're having with just the two of you. Are there new things you've been meaning to try? New skills or toys you want to pick up? There are a lot of ways to add novelty and excitement to your sex life without adding other people. Remembering—and practicing—those things will help make a threesome one more fun thing on the list to try, rather than the only adventure you can have.

If you're going to use dating apps or websites, how much time are you going to spend on them? How many times a week will you log on, and how long will each session last? With the wide array of online options these days, looking for a third for dates could become a full-time job.

Make agreements about how much time you want to dedicate to this project and make sure it stays fun. If it feels like it's eating into your time together, it might be time to take a little step back.

Relationship Agreements

If you have an existing partnership—anything from play partners to spouses—there are agreements. Oftentimes they're unspoken, which is a great way to get into trouble.

Before playing with a third person, it's important to sit down and figure out what your relationship agreements are, or what they need to be, to make multi-person play feel safe and fun.

Here are some things to consider:

▶ Safer-sex boundaries.

▶ Sex acts that are/aren't on the table.

▶ Pet names that are special to the relationship.

▶ Check-ins before play.

▶ Reconnection after play.

> ▶ Overnights with new people.

> ▶ Seeing the same person more than once.

> ▶ Seeing someone separately (outside of the threesome context).

Be sure you understand what your relationship structure is. Do you consider yourselves monogamous, but sometimes play with other people together? Do you think of yourselves as swingers? Are you polyamorous?[3]

Not only will having clarity on structure help avoid hurt feelings down the line, but this is likely a question potential thirds will have for you as well. Some people will want a threesome to be a one-off, or maybe an occasional, casual thing. Others will only be interested if there's a potential relationship component, whether it's a full triad/thrupple, or something else.

If your agreement is that you're only playing together, stick to that. If you want to renegotiate, that requires a conversation. Meeting someone as a couple and then just one of you reaching out to the third is poor form if it wasn't talked about in advance, and it might creep the third out. Not only that, it could be considered cheating by your partner, if that's not what everyone had signed up for.

When you're making agreements, it's a good idea to talk about the possibility of them changing. What you think you need and want when you're starting this process is likely very different from what you'll need a few months or years into it.

People often tell me that the things they thought would be a problem were fine, and issues they never anticipated ended up bothering them. (I had no problem when my ex-husband started

---

3   Check out the glossary for definitions of these structures, and the resource section for books to learn more.

dating or having sex with other people, but I got jealous when he went out to sushi with his new girlfriend. Go figure!)

Remember, too, that agreements can't replace being grown-ass adults. You'll need to use common sense and empathy, and have each other's feelings and best interests in mind. Agreements can be broken—both the letter of the agreement and the spirit. So make sure you're entering into the process in good faith.

Have a Practice Negotiation

Before you bring another actual person into the mix, have a trial run of your negotiation. Talk about celebrities or public figures as your potential threesome partner. Can you agree on who it would be? This is a great chance to take your attractions on a trial run and see where they overlap.

Next, negotiate everything about the theoretical threesome. Which activities are on the table and which are not? Where would you meet up? How would you have the conversations? When the threesome happened, how would it go?

This might sound like a silly exercise, but it's a good way to check for potential problem areas before you run into them with a person in real life. See if there are areas of the conversation where someone is getting jealous, or where you disagree. It's also a way to discover where comparisons or insecurities are lurking.

See how each of you feel when talking about the potential third. When there's an actual person in mind—even if it's someone you'll never meet in real life—it can feel a lot more real than the hypothetical threesome buddy you've been calling to mind so far.

How to Avoid the Pitfalls of *Unicorn Hunting*

Time for some terminology: in the most typically discussed threesome scenario, a *unicorn* is a single, attractive, bisexual woman who will show up to have a threesome with a (likely heterosexual) couple to fulfill their fantasy and then will go away—never to bother them or their relationship again. This magical creature is called a unicorn because they don't exist. All humans have feelings and needs. The term *pegasus* has also been jokingly coined as the male counterpart to the unicorn.

So, if we've got unicorns, what do we call the couples that go looking for them? You guessed it: unicorn hunters.

If you've scrolled through any of the dating apps, you've run across people who say things like, "no couples," or "not your unicorn," in their profile. And while threesomes certainly aren't everybody's cup of tea, this strong aversion is due to a few bad actors. Women who appear to fit the profile of "unicorn" get dozens of propositions online, so these people may already feel objectified.

The theme of this book is treating people with kindness and respect. And when you approach a potential third without any show of interest in who they are as a person, or what they desire, you're not going to get very far. (And rightfully so!)

A disconnect seems to happen for some people when seeking to fulfill a particular kink or sexual fantasy. Even people who would usually be respectful on dating apps begin by talking about what kind of sex they want, before any small talk. It's as though, once they've entered the sex or kink mindset, they forget they're still dealing with real people, rather than fantasy fulfillment robots.

Even if your only goal is a threesome, and you don't plan to have an ongoing relationship with your third, you still need to treat them like a person.

Here are some ways you can do that.

Remember that not everyone who fits your criteria is into couples. Especially if their profile doesn't specify that they're game, sending a message is taking a risk. Do your best to be friendly and polite and don't assume that they're into threesomes (especially not just because they're a bisexual woman/femme.) Not only do you want to represent yourselves well, but ideally your behavior can be so exemplary that it will start to destigmatize couples looking for thirds.

Represent yourselves, and what you're looking for, honestly. Don't be overly vague or make it sound like you're looking for a long-term triad relationship if that's not what you want. If you're interested primarily in a sexy times play partner—say so! I promise, there are people who are into it. And those people will appreciate your candor.

No bait and switch! Represent yourselves as a couple from the get-go. It's not ethical to have what looks like a single's profile and get someone interested, only to spring on them that you're a package deal.

Don't exotify queerness. While exploring sexuality is a perfectly valid reason to be interested in threesomes, make sure not to treat your potential queer partner as a tour guide or someone who will initiate you into a secret queer society. Also, keep in mind the power dynamics at play. Someone who moves through the world as a queer person has doubtless encountered everything from homophobia to discrimination based on their identity. So, to then be objectified for that very identity is deeply hurtful.

Get to know them! Find out what they're interested in—and not just in bed. What are their hobbies? Their favorite books or movies? You need to build some rapport before you jump to the sex talk. And when it comes to sex, you still need to find out what makes them tick. What do they like about threesomes? What are their desires for the encounter?

Even if you've gone into the idea of a threesome with a particular fantasy in mind, make sure there's room for everyone to have their desires fulfilled. If you're describing your fantasy and realize there's no space for taking turns as the center of attention, there may not be much in it for your third. Are you only inviting someone into your fantasy, or are you asking how you can fulfill their desires? Someone else's ideas might be hot, so don't miss out by not asking!

What About Other Couples?

You're reading this book because you're interested in threesomes. The thing is, a lot of people are interested in threesomes. And there are a lot more couples looking than there are single folks. Which is all to say, maybe consider the possibility of playing with other couples as well.

When considering this option, it's important to return to the list of reasons you're interested in having a threesome. If some of those reasons are about exploration and sexual variety, it's possible that a couple could fit the bill just as well as an individual—in fact, with four people you've got even more possible combinations than with three.

Setting your sights on couples rather than singles isn't a magic bullet. Couples aren't simply going to land in your lap (or your bed). And it's worth noting that with more people, there are even more variables when it comes to making sure everyone likes each other and shares some amount of attraction. (Read more about group sex later on.)

Many times couples will form a long-term play arrangement and become friends as well as sex partners. If you're going to play together many times, a number of combinations and scenarios may be possible—as well as potentially breaking off into three-somes occasionally—as long as the odd person out feels good about this exchange. (It helps if there's a rotation of who the three are, and who's at home having movie night for one.)

Read on to learn more about threesomes, but keep this option in the back of your mind. If finding singles proves difficult, or you happen to run into other curious couples on your threesome journey, give this option another thought.

Seeing a Professional

If you live in an area where sex work is legal, you may want to consider hiring a professional. For many of the same reasons that a visit to a strip club can be helpful, hiring a professional can make for very tidy boundaries. You don't need to worry about online personal ads or in-person pickup lines, you can simply be direct about what you want.

Just like at a strip club, remember that everyone must be treated with kindness and respect—whether they're on the clock or not. Paying someone for their time doesn't exempt you from treating someone well, or negotiating and respecting boundaries. According to Dr. Nerdlove, "If you're interested in as uncomplicated a threesome as you can find, an escort is likely your best bet."[v]

Another professional option would be to hire a stripper to come to your home for a private show. If you already tried the strip club exploration, maybe you had a favorite dancer or two you could ask.

Having them come to your home has a few benefits. Firstly, you don't have the distraction of the club environment. And secondly, if having the private show gets you all revved up, you and your sweetie are right by your bedroom if you want to act on all that arousal as soon as your dancer guest leaves—rather than having to navigate the trip home from a club first.

If you go with this option, expect to pay first and tip well. And don't expect different rules to apply just because you're at home. There's still no touching without permission—and don't count on getting it.

Face Your Fears

One of the most powerful discoveries about openness in a relationship is the way it actually reinforces and strengthens the relationship. People sometimes lean on monogamy based on the belief that it keeps them safe from loss. I get it, I've got my own deep seated fears of loss to deal with.

But counting on monogamy for that security isn't a sure thing. Despite agreements, people cheat. People leave.

This isn't much of a pep talk yet, is it?

What I'm getting at is that wanting monogamy for the sake of security is like relying on having a monopoly to keep your business strong. But how secure is a choice if it's not really a choice?

What can be really powerful is if someone has all the options in the world, and they still choose you. *That* feels amazing.

While it can take an incredible leap of faith, sharing a partner with someone else and seeing that it doesn't diminish their love or lust for you is incredibly reaffirming. It's a firsthand way of seeing that they aren't with you because of a lack of options, but because of genuine desire.

You can get these benefits in many ways—maybe it's a one-time threesome or maybe you'll dive into full-fledged multi-person relationships such as polyamory. Whatever you choose, think about how powerful it might be to see someone desiring you, reaching for you, even when someone else is right there.

8

UNICORN TIPS

A Unicorn Tale

When my marriage opened up and I got on the dating apps for the first time (they'd come of age while I was in a period of monogamy), one of the first things I did was proudly (and optimistically) label myself as a unicorn in my dating profile bio.

For me, at that time, the term unicorn seemed to capture the spirit of free and easy exploration I was looking for. And I seemed to fit most of the criteria. A bisexual woman who, given my marriage, wasn't looking for a nesting relationship. It seemed like an ideal way to get back into having new sexual adventures for the first time in roughly a decade.

Unfortunately, I didn't yet know what I was doing, and after several disappointing conversations and one disappointing drinks date I changed my bio and focused on solo dating for a while.

My experience mirrors that of many self-identified unicorns. Not just in the disappointing part, but in that I didn't know what I was doing.

While I still occasionally refer to myself as a unicorn in a tongue-in-cheek way, it seems that many who self-identify that way on dating apps are new to the scene. The reason to worry about this is that it can make you a target for some less than wholesome types who are looking to take advantage of people who might not know better yet.

How you decide to identify is a personal decision, but remember that dating apps and websites are a social experiment, and if you're not getting the results you're looking for, you can change variables and see how that changes your experience. You can always try a version of your profile with "unicorn" in it and one without, and see how that changes the kinds of messages you're getting.

Luckily for me, I began running in kinky and polyamorous circles and ended up having opportunities for threesomes and group sex through the new group of friends I was making. It was much easier to connect in that way with people I already had some rapport with.

After a few years of that, and with many threesomes under my belt, I finally revisited the idea of using apps to meet couples, with much more success.

Why Unicorn?

While I've heard a lot of singles—especially single, bisexual women—scoff at the idea of being a "unicorn," there are also lots of people who quite enjoy the experience. And I'm one of them. When done well, there's something really lovely about getting to be the guest star and then going home to your own bed and your own life.

It can be like taking a little vacation into someone else's relationship—and when the couple is kind and loving, that can be quite a treat. It's also lovely to be part of an encounter where everyone is incredibly grateful that you're there. And the unicorn often gets to be the star of the show. After all, you're the one making this fantasy come true.

Here are some potential benefits of being a unicorn:

▸ The couple is often *very* happy you're there. That kind of gratitude is good for anyone's ego.

▸ You get to have the benefits of hot threesome sex without the risk of relationship fallout. (Of course, this book is trying to reduce that risk, but it's still a possibility.)

▸ As they say, many hands make light work. So if you'd usually be a little worried about performing for a new partner, in a threesome that task is shared.

▸ The best of both worlds? If you happen to be bisexual or pansexual, and you're joining a couple of mixed genders, it can be a nice treat to explore multiple sides of your attractions at once.

In the following pages we'll explore how to find existing couples for threesomes, how to figure out if they're the right fit for you, and how to make sure your fantasies and desires get equal weight and consideration while negotiating and playing.

How To Go Couple Hunting

While you could certainly try what I did and advertise yourself as a unicorn, that method can backfire. It's likely to get a lot of attention, and maybe not the kind you want.

These days I prefer a more subtle approach. I might say something like "open to singles and couples" somewhere in a dating app profile, or I might just make the first move myself when I see a couple's profile that catches my eye.

The apps are becoming ever more friendly to couples' profiles—from shared profiles on OKCupid to apps that cater to couples or open relationships.[4] When you're looking at a profile, does it seem balanced, or is it mostly one person in all the pictures? Are the pictures overtly sexual, or are you seeing some of the people's hobbies and personalities too? Are they showing their faces or just their bodies? Or, are all the pictures memes and images stolen from the internet? If you've never been on dating apps before, it can take some time to get comfortable. But once you do, you'll learn to get a feel for people pretty quickly.

Chapter 11 will list places to meet people for threesomes, and all of those places apply to unicorns, too. If you're eyeing couples at a party or mixer, check out their interactions with each other. Make sure it seems like they're in this together. And read on for more about what to look for.

How To Screen a Couple

While attraction and chemistry are important, the number one thing to pay attention to when meeting a couple is how they're interacting with each other. Are they getting along and communicating well? Are they checking in with each other? Do they seem in tune with each other's needs? These are all great signs.

On the other hand, if one person seems way more into it than the other, or if one person is doing all of the talking, I get nervous. All too often the threesome is one person's fantasy and the other is just along for the ride, and this can spell trouble. You never want to end up involved in sex with someone who doesn't really want to be there.

Beyond both seeming on board with the idea, do they both seem interested in you? Depending how sexualities align, do you feel like you're being flirted with by both parties? Chemistry is

---

4   See resources in the back for options as of this printing, but keep in mind the online dating world evolves quickly. Many apps disappear and new ones are always being created.

important, so look for the same spark you'd be looking for on a date with just one person.

If you're potentially interested but not sure about chemistry or attraction, suggest a hang out first. Maybe you all get coffee or do some activity together. It'll give you more of a chance to see if you're all attracted to each other. And you'll also be able to find out how serious the couple is. If there're not willing to put a little time into getting to know you, then they may not have your interests and desires in mind.

As you're hanging out, in whatever context, make sure you ask any screening questions you'd normally ask before a sexual encounter. And on top of that, come up with a few threesome-specific questions, too.

I like to know if the people involved have had a threesome before. Not that it has to be a deal-breaker if they haven't—but it can be a little riskier if one or both people don't know how they'll handle things in the moment. Maybe unexpected jealousy or comparison will pop up, or maybe the couple will even have a threesome-inspired conflict. Just be ready to remove yourself from the situation if at any point it stops feeling comfortable.

You might also want to know why the couple is interested in having a threesome. Like with all sex, there are countless possible motivations—and having motivations aligned between all parties is one important step for having great sex.

Speaking of sex, once you're having more explicit conversations, you might want to ask what their number one threesome desire is. Maybe there's a particular position or sex act they're dying to try. If their number one kink isn't your jam, then it's worth finding out if they're willing to skip it, or if this simply isn't a good fit. And the same goes for you—if there's anything you absolutely need as part of a threesome for it to feel worth it, it's worth checking in advance to see if they're interested.

Similarly, it's worth asking about their boundaries and limits. Some couples might have a rule against kissing or overnights, for example. If that's fine with you, go for it! But if that's going to make you feel less respected as a person or a partner, then maybe it's not a great fit.

Keep in mind that you shouldn't be the only one asking questions! One thing to look for is whether the couple seems interested in you as a person, and interested in what you're hoping to get from the experience. If you're just being used to fulfill a fantasy then the experience might not go very far towards meeting your needs—unless fulfilling couples' fantasies is your kink.

If I'm on a first date with a couple and going home together that night is a possibility, I like to take a bathroom break as an excuse to leave them alone together. If I'm going home with them, I want to make absolutely sure they've had a chance to check in with each other without me watching to see if they're both on board.

If you want, you can even announce that's what you're doing. Say, "I'm going to step outside and check my phone so you two can talk about me." It can be playful and true at the same time.

It can also be a good chance for you to do a gut-check. When face to face with people, it's easy to go with the flow, but having a moment alone to listen to yourself can be valuable to make sure you're really feeling it and not just being polite.

If spur of the moment decisions don't feel right for you, it can be helpful to set a policy for yourself that first dates are just screening meetings. Then, if everyone clicks, you can make a second date to have sex. That way everyone gets a solid chance to think things over, sleep on it, and make sure it's really the right fit for everyone involved—rather than giving into any pressure in the moment.

Advocating for Yourself

A lot of the language we have around threesomes, including the term *unicorn* itself, centers an existing couple in the experience. It's their fantasy, and a third is coming in just to meet the couple's needs.

But a good threesome doesn't have to be that way. Going into a threesome with a good idea of your desires, and the ability to advocate for yourself, goes a long way towards creating a pleasurable experience.

If you're joining an existing couple, there's a good chance they've been fantasizing about, and talking about, this threesome for a long time. They have ideas for how they'd like it to go, what positions they want to try, and what they're hoping to get out of it.

At this point you've hopefully already screened for whether their fantasies leave room for your pleasure—but even with that step, it helps to feel confident advocating for yourself and your needs.

What are *you* hoping to get out of this experience? Do you like the idea of being the star of the show and the center of attention? Are you excited about experiencing a new dynamic or learning a new skill?

If you're curious about exploring your sexuality, a threesome can be a nice way to dip your toes in the water. You can find a couple with a person of the gender you want to explore with, and a person of a gender you're already familiar with. This can feel like safer footing for trying something new.

You can also advocate for the logistics that will make you the most comfortable. Do you want to be at your place or at theirs? You might feel more comfortable on your home turf, but leaving someone else's house is easier than throwing people out of yours. Consider the pros and cons of the options.

If you don't want an overnight, it's helpful to state an end time at the beginning. But whether or not the end is prearranged, you can always leave whenever you want to.

What needs do you have for right after sex or for the days that follow? Be sure to speak up about those needs, commonly called *aftercare*, as well. If you know you'll want a check-in the next day by text, or even a get-together, make sure the couple is on board. Everyone has different expectations around aftercare and follow up, so it's a good idea to make sure you're in alignment.

Red and Yellow Flags

Many of the things that give *unicorn hunters* a bad name are due to lack of experience, rather than ill intent. But that doesn't make them any more fun to deal with. The good news is that simple lack of information is a very solvable problem.

If you're interacting with a couple and something gets your hackles up, you need to decide if that's a sign that you should just be out of there, or if there's something you'd like to talk through with them.

To make this determination, think about:

▶ How excited are you about this particular couple?

▶ Do they seem open and willing to learn?

▶ Are they taking your feelings and concerns seriously?

As the saying goes, there are plenty of fish in the sea. And if you're a single person looking to play with a couple, you have the advantage of numbers on your side. So if a particular situation doesn't feel right, don't hesitate to move on and find other people to play with. With that in mind, here are some things to think about and watch out for.

★ ★ ★

Is the couple being clear and straightforward about what they're looking for?

Unfortunately, some couples seem to think that offering a long-term relationship or triad situation is more likely to get them dates than being upfront about wanting a threesome. So, if you're specifically wanting a long-term arrangement, do enough talking and hanging out to make sure everyone is on the same page. Plenty of people are interested in triads, it's just a few bad actors making that seem like a shady pickup line.

How does hierarchy play out in their relationship?

Many couples who are looking for a threesome are interested in a shared adventure while still prioritizing their existing relationship—and that's okay! What's important to look for is how they're framing this priority.

If there's a lot of language about the relationship coming first, it could be a sign that there are some insecurities that may lead to unfair treatment of the third. Like in many dating scenarios, you'll have to trust your gut and see if what they're describing seems like something you're excited to be part of.

Are you being presented with a list of rules?

Many couples will have established boundaries about what they are and aren't okay with during a threesome. And boundaries are good! Having well-thought-out limits and boundaries is a great sign that the couple has done their homework and is up for the communication needed to negotiate a threesome. But if the boundaries are expressed as a list of rules for you, the third, to follow, that's a potential problem. (For more discussion on the difference between rules and boundaries, see Chapter 14.)

Rules are often put in place as a (misguided) attempt to address someone's fears or insecurities. So look out for these kinds of rules as a potential red flag for future trouble. For instance, if a couple states that the third can't engage in kissing with the couple—maybe the no kissing rule is an attempt to legislate against jealousy, or the possibility of romantic feelings developing.

Because these kind of rules rarely have their desired effect, it's likely the jealous or insecure partner will still be uncomfortable in the moment, and that might cause some friction. And while jealousy and insecurity are totally normal things to feel, they should be addressed as much as possible in advance. If they need to be addressed in the moment, it should be with kindness for everyone involved.

9

THREESOME INTERLUDE

The Threesome That Didn't Happen (Yet)

I'm sure you've heard the saying that real life is stranger than fiction? The thing with fiction is that you can tie things up with a tidy bow. Real life tends to be messy.

I do a lot of live storytelling shows, so I'm always pulling from my real life for stories to tell on stage. And it can be tricky to find a tidy narrative arc in things that have really happened.

There's one story I've wanted to tell, but I've never been able to use it because it doesn't have a satisfying ending. Finally that story finds a home here—because in the context of this book, the lack of an ending is the point.

People in my generation got to have an interesting experience of losing touch with people after high school and college, and then finding them again once social media sites started coming online. I got to have this experience, too.

Maybe ten years after graduation, I heard from someone I'd dated in high school. While the relationship hadn't been serious, it left an impact on me. So I was thrilled to hear from him again. However, at this point I was married (monogamously, at the time) and we lived on different sides of the country.

We renewed our friendship and wrote back and forth to each other on a regular basis. To be honest, it probably pushed the boundaries of platonic friendship. But, I justified, it was long distance. We weren't actually going to see each other.

Time passed. Our lives changed.

He got married. My marriage opened up. Then I got divorced. More time passed.

Then one day I got a message from him. Their relationship was open now too, and he wondered if I'd be interested in a threesome.

At this point we hadn't spent time in person together since high school. And we'd never had sex. But I was intrigued. By now I was deep into the various sexuality communities in my area, and threesomes were a standard part of my life. And who isn't curious about the one who got away, with the added bonus of his beautiful wife!

We sent messages back and forth talking about the possibility. What would it look like? How would it work? I'd have to fly out to see them, but they have a guest room, so no pressure, he said.

In general, I'm hesitant about participating in a first threesome (or a first anything) because the stakes are so high. But I was so curious about him, and it would be such a tidy end to our story.

But then I got a message from his wife. And while it was perfectly friendly, and she seemed up for the threesome idea, the things she was saying just didn't perfectly line up with what he'd told me. I was worried that they weren't on the same page, and feared I'd be wading into some kind of mess. So I had to pass.

But these days they have a lot more experience . . . so maybe by the time this book gets a second edition, we'll have finally gotten together for our threesome. A sexual adventure decades in the making.

HOW DO
SEXUALITIES ALIGN?

How Will People Combine?

One of the things you need to think about when planning a threesome is what kind of interactions you want between the people involved. A threesome doesn't have to be a free-for-all between all parties. Maybe it's a *V*-shaped arrangement, with one person the center of attention. This could be for any number of reasons, from relationship agreements, to sexualities and attraction, to some of the participants having a more platonic connection.

So, when thinking about combinations, decide what kind of connections you're hoping to have, in order to inform partner choice, and then negotiate with the individuals in question to see if desires and attractions align.

While my general preference in threesomes is for everyone to be into everyone, sometimes it's nice to be the center of attention. It can also simplify the negotiation, as well as the position choice. And remember, there are different ways to be "into" someone. At a minimum, everyone should be comfortable together and friendly. But that can happen without everyone kissing or engaging in sexual touch.

In a recent threesome I had with two men, I simply asked them, "Are you interested in interacting with each other, or do you both want to focus on me?" I knew both of the men to be open to play with other men, but that's no guarantee they were attracted to each other. They also didn't know each other very well. I was the connection between the two. Because of this, I also took the lead on negotiation.

I was on a date with one of the men, and the other was a friend and occasional play partner. We were at a play party, which made it easy to transition from flirting to negotiating to playing. We simply moved from a social area to a small room with a bed (but no door, so people could watch.)

To help with sexual safety, the men wore gloves when fingering me, and wore condoms for oral and vaginal sex. We ended up in the *spit-roast* position, which you'll read about in a few chapters, and aside from a high five over my back at my encouragement, the fellas didn't really make much contact.

Even so, it was a playful encounter for everyone, with the men chatting and joking, and everyone finding a place to put a hand, or place a kiss.

Remember that sexuality or identity won't guarantee interest or attraction—or lack thereof. You don't expect all straight men and all straight women to be into each other, so remember it's no more likely that all bisexual people would be into each other, either.

Not only that, but activities and labels don't have to align in any particular way. Someone can identify as straight and still want to explore kissing, touching, or more with someone of the same gender. And the opposite is true, too. So make sure you go into negotiations without making any assumptions about who is up for what. You simply need to ask everyone what they're interested in and give them space to explore.

Don't Fake It

Faking any kind of pleasure is a bad idea. Not only are you not enjoying yourself—hence the faking—but you're misleading the other people involved. I think this is a problem on an ethical level, but it also creates a practical issue—if someone thinks you enjoy something, they're going to keep doing it. That's why faking orgasms is such a problem. You create a loop where someone keeps doing what you don't enjoy, you keep faking it, and you don't get to adjust to something you would enjoy.

With threesomes, sometimes people agree to the adventure just to please a partner. But that's risky and likely to backfire. While maybe you can sit through a movie you're not jazzed about because your partner is into it, that's a far cry from participating in sex you don't want to be having.

It simply isn't good for you to try and do sexy things you're not into. It will create negative associations around sex that can have a lasting impact, and it can build resentment towards your partner that can poison the relationship.

Not only that, but people can tell. A third will know if you're not really into them or aren't excited about them touching your partner. At best it will be awkward, at worst the whole thing will melt down.

Sometimes people say they're game for same-sex action as part of a threesome because they think it's what's expected, even if they're not into it. Same as above, this is a bad idea.

It's one thing to be unsure and curious. Simply let the people involved know that this is an experiment for you and you might need to stop.

But if you *know* you're not into it, don't just grit your teeth and play along. There are plenty of ways to have a threesome that don't include all parties doing all the things with everyone. So find ways to participate that stay well within your comfort zone, and everyone will have a much better time.

The bottom line is that it isn't fair to you, or to anyone else involved, to engage in any forms of sex or play you're not enthusiastic about.

Here's what one woman had to say:

> Don't have sex with a couple unless you want to have sex with BOTH of them: a cautionary tale.
>
> Once I had a big crush on a girl I worked with. She was voluptuous, with curly long raven hair and a sly smile. We flirted a bit, but I was young and a #newqueer so I didn't know how to make the first move. Eventually she asked me out for drinks. I was so excited, I bought a new dress for the occasion. When I got there, my stomach dropped when I saw a man with her, her boyfriend.
>
> I figured I had misunderstood the signals. Disappointing, but I decided to just go with it. We all played pool, and I eventually suggested we go to the lesbian bar, hoping I could meet someone there. When we got there, we all got a little drunk, and then it became apparent to me what was happening.
>
> All of a sudden I was being grinded on by her boyfriend in the back and her in the front. We started kissing, so I let him do whatever he was doing back there, I was just so thrilled to be kissing her.
>
> We eventually moved to their hot tub, where I continued to focus on her—he penetrated me without checking in, and kept gnawing at my breasts. The sex we had was fine, but I felt constantly annoyed by his presence.

The Assumptions

If you're googling around or looking for stock photos of three-somes, you're likely to find a man with two women. (Likely all cisgendered, white, and thin, too.) This hardly represents the infinite range of combinations a threesome can include. Still, a threesome is one of the most common fantasies among hetero-sexual or heterosexual-leaning couples, so this combination is one of the most common.

Why is the third more often depicted as a woman? All too often, men in relationships think the idea of their partner with another woman is hot, while the idea of her with another man is out of the question. Add to that our culture's prevailing homophobia, and you've got a recipe for FMF threesomes.

And there's certainly nothing wrong with that alignment of people. Just remember how easy it is to get into trouble when you're making assumptions rather than explicit negotiations. And make sure everything about who is included and how they're interacting gets discussed well in advance.

Other Gender and Sexuality Configurations

Any combination of three people you can imagine can have a threesome!

Be careful about using exclusionary or fetishizing language when looking for a couple or a third for your threesome. While you may have a particular combination of people in mind, there are lots of options, so don't make the mistake of thinking other people have the same assumptions as you.

The best threesomes embrace the spirit of exploration, so take a close look at what assumptions you're making and pick those assumptions apart. When you sat down and thought about why you wanted to have a threesome—what were your answers? And are those answers gender dependent? There's a good chance most of the things you want can happen with any combination of people.

No, All Women Aren't Bi

Through a combination of mediocre science, bad media interpretations of that science, and general cultural assumptions, people seem to assume all women are bisexual, or at least heteroflexible.

Let's dig into this science a bit.

The recent study[vi] that led to a flurry of these overly simplistic headlines measured arousal by monitoring vaginal lubrication or blood flow in women and level of erection in men. Research of this kind often receives criticism for including only cisgendered people, ignoring trans and nonbinary identities. Not only that, but lubrication to erection is not an apples-to-apples methodology.[vii]

Those problems aside, what the study found was that women tend to respond to "sexually relevant stimuli" across a wide range of images. For example, pictures of men together, women together, and even animals.

At the same time that they were checking in with the genitals, the study participants had a dial to turn in order to indicate their subjective arousal—meaning whether or not they were into the image they were seeing.

The difference between what our brains are thinking and what our genitals are doing is referred to as *arousal nonconcordance*. For example, if a woman experienced increased vaginal lubrication or blood flow while looking at an image, but her mental response was one of no interest in the image, that would be described as arousal nonconcordance.

In Emily Nagoski's *Come As You Are*, she summarizes this research as showing a roughly 50% agreement between genital response and subjective arousal for men, and only 10% for women.

Unfortunately, the media hot take was that women are turned on by everything—which is absolutely not true. A better take would be that genital response often isn't in alignment with actual interest, so we have to believe what people tell us—imagine that!

This means that being wet or hard isn't the same as being turned on, and being dry or soft isn't the same as being turned off. This can be a difficult reframe, because we often use the words *hard* or *wet* as a stand-in for saying someone was turned on.

Another study[viii] conducted by the CDC found that more than 5% of women identified as bisexual, versus roughly 2% of men. Right off the bat, you need to be suspicious of any self-reporting survey, as there is always a cultural bias to consider.

In this case, it's impossible to separate cultural stigma against bisexuality when it comes to self-reporting. The lower number of men identifying as bisexual could be influenced by greater stigma against bisexual men, as well as greater homophobia directed at men. While on the flip side, bisexuality in women (at least in a performative way) is often encouraged.

What does this mean for you?

Never make assumptions about someone's sexuality or their turn-ons. Be sure to explicitly ask what people enjoy. You'll likely get a lot of valuable information.

Don't assume that all women are up for girl-on-girl action. Or that women are naturally any more flexible in their sexuality than men are. (Or people of other genders, for that matter.)

You should also know that there isn't an out bi woman on the planet who hasn't been propositioned for a threesome. Maybe even more times than she can count. It tends to be people's go-to response when hearing about your identity. So even when a woman does self-identify as bisexual, remember that doesn't necessarily mean she's into threesomes, and it certainly doesn't mean she's automatically interested in a threesome with you. So follow all the guidelines here about treating people with respect, and you'll have much better chances.

Considerations with Two Straight Men

While the culture is beginning to shift, many people grew up surrounded by homophobia, and that can make the idea of being naked in a sexual space with another man feel a little fraught. Not only that, but depending on the positions you're choosing, there may be some close contact between two men. With some positions (double penetration, etc.) there may even be genital to genital contact.

You probably already know if you're completely against any of the above—but what about if you're not sure? If you're still figuring out how you feel about the situation, be sure to go slowly. Set clear boundaries and let everyone involved know that you're exploring your feelings and may need to slow down or stop.

From people who've talked to me about their experiences, it often seems to work better if the men involved are already friends. The threesome can even function as a platonic bonding experience, and this works especially well if the overall tone of the experience is playful. (Look for positions later on that include a jovial high five.)

For folks who engage in open relationships, a likely combination is a woman with two men who are already her partners. In this case, the men are hopefully already at least friendly with each other, if not friends. And the existing rapport with the woman can help ease any potential discomfort.

If you're looking for a third man for an MFM threesome, where the men won't be sexually involved with each other, you still want the fellas to get along. So even if you're starting with a stranger you've met online, for example, you want everyone to meet up and make sure they enjoy each other's company.

Here's what John Strange had to say,

> *I am attracted enough to men to admire their sexiness at a short distance, but not enough that kissing them stops feeling awkward and unsatisfying. (Why bother when there are WOMEN in the world?) In a threesome with a woman and another man, the heat of my interaction with her thins the wall of heterosexuality just enough that the inherent awkwardness of being naked and aroused with another man disappears, because she can be the focus of my energy, and he and I are aligned rather than interacting together.*
>
> *Plus, I have a very strong voyeuristic impulse. Even with a mirror there are limits to how well I can watch my lover when I am having sex with them. In a threesome, I get to see a lover deep in her passion in a way I cannot otherwise.*

If you're going to negotiate an MFM threesome where the guys keep their distance from each other, be careful of the language you use to negotiate that. I've heard people say, half joking, "no gay stuff." While that might sound harmless, remember that you don't know where the other person is coming from, and this can easily offend. Not to mention the offense you may give to anyone else within ear shot. If you don't want sexual contact with someone, that's always your choice to make, but be sure to make your preference known in a respectful way.

It's also worth remembering that actions don't dictate identity. There are no "straight police" who will come and take your straight card away if they find out you were naked with another guy, or even kissed or went down on another guy.

This behavior is in fact so common that there have been sociological studies done on the phenomenon. A 2018 article in the *Journal of Sexualities* discusses it thusly,

> *Based on their patterns of sexual interpretation, we discuss how these men make their same-sex desires and behaviours consistent with a primary self-identification as straight. We argue that, in the process of maintaining identities as straight men, they change the definition of heterosexuality, in effect turning it into a considerably elastic category that is perceived as fully compatible with having and enacting same-sex desires.[ix]*

Or, to paraphrase, a heterosexual or straight identity doesn't have to be a tight box you find yourself in. You always get to choose how you identify, regardless of what behaviors you engage in. In fact, many straight men may choose to have these explorations with other straight men because of the safety they feel in that shared identity.

11

HOW TO MEET
PEOPLE FOR THREESOMES

Becoming a Threesome Person

There's an episode of the TV series *Seinfeld* that's a prime example of sitcom relationship logic. In the episode, Seinfeld's friend, Costanza, advises that, instead of being direct and breaking up with someone, Seinfeld should propose a threesome so his girl-friend will be offended and break up with him.

Then comes the scene that has stayed with me for life, that I regularly quote to myself, for my own amusement. Seinfeld tells Costanza that the plan didn't work because, "She's into it . . . and the roommate is into it too."[x]

Constanza equates this to discovering plutonium by acci-dent—because, of course, everyone is supposed to consider a threesome the ultimate goal.

But Seinfeld says he can't do it, because he's not an "orgy guy." He says that if he were going to do it he'd need to change everything about himself, going on to itemize the way orgy guys behave, with special outfits, new toiletries, different furniture, and perhaps my favorite, "new friends—orgy friends."

And while this is all meant to be a punchline, because people who participate in any non-normative sex are an easy target, there's a bit of truth to it. Goodness knows there are no shortage of robes or lotions in my house, and I do put special thought into my bedspreads and lighting.

Of course, having a threesome or two doesn't mean you need a whole new lifestyle and whole new friend group. But you may find that running in "orgy guy" circles does make threesomes more likely.

While there are people who seemingly trip and fall into threesomes on a regular basis, there are others who have been desperate for threesomes for years and can't seem to make it happen. Some of it is a matter of luck, and some of it depends on other factors, like the culture in the city or town where you live. But a lot of it comes down to the lifestyle and friend groups that you cultivate.

If you are actively part of sex-positive, open-relationship, and kink communities, you're going to have a lot more access to the people and places that make threesomes more likely to happen. If you're part of a monogamous couple, have mostly monogamous friends, and aren't active in any sex-based communities, it's going to be a little trickier to get started.

The good news is that all of this is ultimately under your control. The question is how much time and energy you want to put into making a threesome happen—especially if you're interested in a one-off more than a lifestyle.

So what now? Start by talking to your friends. You might be surprised to learn they're more sexually adventurous than you'd realized. It's possible you already have an in to these communities and just didn't know it.

Aside from the crowd you run with, there are other ways to become a "threesome person," and they're all well within reach.

▶ For starters, become well acquainted with sexual safety, testing, barrier use, and having safer-sex talks.

▶ Become adept at communication—communicating your own desires and boundaries, as well as ways to check in with the other people involved.

▶ Think critically about your interactions and expectations to ensure that you treat people like people, not like sex toys or threesome vending machines.

What else does it mean to be a threesome person, or an orgy guy? Think about all the qualities you're hoping for in a threesome partner or partners. You're probably hoping for someone who is a good communicator. Someone who doesn't have a lot of "drama" in their life. Someone who is good at boundaries and also has a wide and varied sexual skill set. Am I on the right track?

Remember that these awesome lovers with good boundaries are also going to be screening *you*. So if you want them to judge you threesome worthy, try to become all of these things yourself.

Keep all of this in mind as you try to meet someone new for a threesome. If you burn out on online dating or trying to meet a stranger, circle back to this conversation. Decide how badly you want to have a threesome. If you want it badly enough, it might be worth a lifestyle shift.

Becoming a Threesome Couple

The following pages are going to tell you about places you can go and things you can do to try and find partners for your threesome fantasy. But the number one most effective way to find a third is to be the kind of couple a third would want to be with.

We just talked about some ways to be a threesome person—and those all apply to the individuals in a couple. But what else?

Make sure you two actually *like* each other. I've gotten a surprising number of couples in my office who filled out intake forms saying they want to explore threesomes or open relationships or kink, and then they sit at the opposite ends of the couch and don't make eye contact.

I've said it before, and I'll say it again. If you're having problems in your relationship, a threesome is not the solution. Work on the relationship first, then level up to new adventures when you two are solid.

I say this not only because a threesome, should you line one up, will likely backfire for you two if your relationship isn't solid. But because your third will be able to tell. You probably won't be able to find a third person, and if you do, they probably won't last long.

You want to move into this process feeling solid and confident in your relationship. Because that's going to show as you're out mingling and mixing. That's the dynamic that thirds will want to be part of.

When you're out at an event together, give each other some space and come together for the occasional check-in. It's important to trust each other enough to do a bit of exploring on your own, and then to come back together and see how each of you are feeling. This confident and secure behavior will be visible to others. And this is what your potential partners want to see.

Laughing, joking, being playful—the elements we're likely to want in an eventual threesome—can be on display while you're out at a party or event. People gravitate to that kind of energy. So if you want to find a third for a threesome, be the couple the third wants to be with.

Avoiding Culture Clash

Going looking for threesome partners is likely to send you into communities you might not be familiar with. In addition to treating people with respect, it's worth learning about the differences in each microculture so you don't accidentally put your foot in your mouth.

If you show up in an online chat room—or public meet-up—and the first things you have to say are what you're looking for, you'll be shut down in just about any community.

But that doesn't mean there isn't a time and a place for the personal ad style approach, it just means you need to get to know people first and become known in whatever community you're joining. If you've only shown up to cruise, you'll be spotted a mile away and likely won't get the time of day.

In swinger culture and at swinger clubs, the vibe is usually very couples-centric. And they're predominantly cisgendered, heterosexual couples. Many events will be only for couples, or for couples and single women. When events are open to everyone, they sometimes explicitly limit the number of single men allowed to attend, or they balance the numbers by charging far more for single men (and the lowest price for single women).

While gender-based pricing isn't my jam, I understand why it's the norm in some of those communities. When the majority of people showing up to play are heterosexual, and couples, they're looking for *gender balance*. If that falls in line with what you're looking for—great! However, if you fall outside of those particular lines, these events might not feel super comfortable for you.

While things vary regionally and even between clubs, swinger events often have some amount of casual touching. Meaning, someone might put a hand on your arm or shoulder while talking to you. Sometimes they'll go even further than that, waiting for a "no" rather than asking for a "yes." Again, these standards aren't my personal preference, but they seem to work for a lot of people. So make sure to read up on what you're getting yourself into, and feel out the space for codes of conduct before getting in too deep.

In swinger spaces, it's also not uncommon for people to play in private rooms with a door open, or even in more public places, if they want someone to join in. Generally, the etiquette here is simply to ask if someone is looking for company. (Always ask first!) If a door is closed, however, people are not to be disturbed.

Kink events tend to be much more strict about consent than swinger parties. While rules can vary, expect there to be no touch whatsoever without asking, and that applies to people's toys, too.

Sometimes kink events will be held in swinger clubs, or other shared venues, and sometimes they will be in dedicated play spaces. If a venue is a full-time dungeon, be prepared to see kink furniture and equipment. Check out the party or venue website to get an idea of what you're walking into.

If the idea of seeing people hitting each other (spanking, flogging, etc.) is a turn-off, these parties probably aren't for you. You're also likely to hear a fair amount of screaming.

Some kink parties allow sex, and some only allow BDSM play, while still others draw arbitrary lines around sex or nudity. I used to help out at one kink party held at a bar that had to follow state laws for bars and restaurants, and that led to many silly rules—like people with penises could be nude, but had to be facing a wall. It's also possible that a party will allow penetration with fingers or toys, but not with a penis.

Depending on the size and culture of the event, people may be mostly playing with folks they know already or had prearranged plans with, or they may be open to pickup play. Keep in mind, though, that at a kink event pickup play may well include only kink activities, not sex. So if you're curious about three-way kink dynamics, or watching a partner get spanked, etc., this could be a good fit.

★ ★ ★

If you're going to polyamory events, they're more likely to be meet-ups in public places and other mixer-type events. These can be great places to meet friends and build community, but they're rarely a good place to actively recruit for partners. Some polyamory communities will host speed-dating events or other similar mixers, and these may be a good fit.

You might also find a variety of queer meet-ups and parties. If you don't identify as queer, or as falling somewhere on the LGBTQ+ spectrum, these events are probably not for you. Showing up only to find a partner is likely to be seen as fetishizing and objectifying and will lead to ill will and no dates.

However, if these labels or identities do apply to you, or to the partner you're hoping to have a threesome with, these events could be a good fit—with caution.

If you're showing up only to cruise, it's not going to work out. Like polyamory meet-ups, queer events are a good chance to make friends and build community—and yes, some of those connections may lead to dates and partners down the line. But these events aren't a good fit if you're looking for instant gratification on the threesome front.

Whatever events you're planning to go to, or communities you're hoping to join, do your research first. Show up in good faith as a participant to the event, and be willing to watch and learn.

What Are You Looking For?

Have you thought about who your ideal threesome buddies are? Whether you're a couple looking for a third, or a solo person looking for one or two others, you'll want to find people who are the best fit for you.

Believe it or not, attraction is the easy part. You know who you're attracted to, or you know it when you see it. But there are other important traits that you can't tell just by looking at somebody. As we talk about negotiations and safer sex talks, we'll go into some detail about what to look for in those conversations—but what about overall traits that make someone a good threesome candidate?

Ideally, you want any sex partner to be good at communication. And that's doubly (triply?) true when it comes to threesomes or any other varsity-level adventure. If someone can't speak up for themselves about what they do or don't want, you're way more likely to run into trouble, either during the threesome itself or afterwards. So only play with people who demonstrate they know what they're getting themselves into and have the language to talk about it.

One example of this to look out for is whether someone demonstrates the ability to say "no." Has the person you're thinking of playing with always agreed to your choice of restaurant, the movie you want to see, and every sex adventure you've proposed? This could be a sign that they haven't figured out their own boundaries or that they have trouble expressing them. And this can spell trouble down the line.

Similar to communication skills, you want to look out for emotional maturity. Can someone talk about sex and body parts without falling into giggles? Sure, some of this stuff is silly or even embarrassing, but it's important that people can say the words if they're going to do the deeds.

When looking for threesome partners, screen for a lot of the same things you would in any dating or hookup scenario. Ask questions about someone's exes, previous sexual adventures, or other threesomes. Watching how people talk about previous partners is a great way to find out how they see people. Sure, we've all had one (or two) relationships that weren't great, but if someone has a long list of horrible exes they want to tell you about, run the other way. And pay attention to the language they're using, too. Calling an ex "crazy" or any other similar term is a bad sign.

Another great way to find out more about a potential partner is by asking what their deal-breakers are. Some people don't want to date smokers or people with certain political views. That's fine, we all have our preferences. But if they start talking about people's bodies, or talking in generally insulting ways about other humans, that's often a bad sign. Trust your gut and the feeling you get about someone.

While at first it may seem tricky to find people to engage in a threesome with you, you'll get the hang of it eventually. And even if partners are feeling scarce, it's not worth compromising on the things that are important to you—you simply won't have a very good time, or you'll run into trouble after playing. So hold out for people you're really excited about.

Existing Friend(s) or Someone New?

When an existing couple starts discussing the idea of a threesome, the question of who to add is usually one of the first that comes up. Generally, people have strong feelings about whether friends, coworkers, or acquaintances should be potential thirds.

Some people feel the most comfortable with people already in their circles. Others don't like the idea of mixing their sex lives with their social or work dynamics. There isn't a right or wrong answer here, it all comes down to personal preference.

The benefit of choosing someone you know is that there may already be some comfort and familiarity. Perhaps you know someone's outlook on relationships is compatible with your own, or you've heard their stories and know they're adventurous. Hanging out before the threesome might also feel easier if you're all at least friendly, as the conversation can flow more smoothly if you have friends, hobbies, or other things in common.

The potential downside of having a threesome with someone in your social circle is that you're going to keep running into them. If you all have an amazing time, maybe that's a bonus. But if things go sideways and there are hurt feelings, it could put a wrench in social plans if they become someone you want to avoid. Another consideration is whether you're looking for a sexy one-off or whether you're open to an ongoing thing. If you want to have sex and never speak of it again, that'll be extra tricky with someone who is already part of your life.

A potential compromise between these scenarios is someone you already know, but who doesn't live local to you. Then you have the benefits of familiarity without worrying about seeing them at every weekly game night.

A long-distance tryst can also mean coupling the adventure with another common desire enhancer—a vacation! Maybe you take a trip to where this third person lives and make a weekend out of it. Plus, being in a hotel room might feel more comfortable for an activity that already feels edgy, so your personal bedroom can remain a sacred space.

Not all friends or acquaintances are equal when it comes to threesome potential. It's worth considering exactly what the relationship is or was. What about exes? A surprising number of people bring an ex back into the mix if there's still chemistry and friendly connection—after all, if you already know the sex works well between you, that's one less variable. But depending on the other person or relationship involved, it might feel emotionally risky to bring a sexual relationship with an ex into play.

It's not at all uncommon for someone to have an office crush—so should that person be a potential threesome buddy? Similar to the considerations of a friend or acquaintance, but significantly multiplied if this is a person you're going to have to see every day for the rest of your time at that job, it might not be worth the risk of making things weird. And this goes doubly if there's a power differential between you at work. Being mindful of these power dynamics is so important that many workplaces (along with schools and universities) have explicit policies against these relationships.

If you're in an open relationship already, are partners' partners fair game? I tried this once (introducing my boyfriend to my girlfriend), and the two hit it off so well I ended up in an accidental triad. Whether you consider that a pro or a con depends on your preferences and relationship philosophies.

There's also a difference between serious relationships and casual play partners. While bringing multiple serious partners together can have consequences, it can actually work quite well if everyone is a more casual sexual partner.

Three Solo Folks

While you're unlikely to line up two separate dates on one of the apps, threesomes do happen between otherwise unattached parties. I see this most commonly at play parties or sex clubs, where you have ample chance to meet people looking for these kinds of experiences. But they can certainly manifest from other group outings or parties at someone's home.

When everyone involved is new to each other, all the negotiations need to be done from scratch. So be sure there's enough of a check-in that everyone is getting their needs met and has established boundaries.

Sometimes a pair of friends might like engaging in a threesome together, with or without sexual contact between them. Check out the considerations for existing dyads (couples) if this applies to you. While some of that advice assumes a romantic partnership, any existing connection will have unique boundaries.

There can also be threesomes between people who are friends or casual acquaintances, but where there are no existing sexual partnerships in the group. Again, these most easily manifest at parties, but if you've got sexually open and adventurous friends, it's also possible to propose a threesome outside of a party context.

Clubs and Public Parties

If you live in or near a city of any size, you probably have access to sex clubs or venues that host sex parties. In smaller or more conservative areas these may be house parties, where you need to know someone to get invited. In Chapter 5 we discussed using parties as a way to dip your toes into exploration—here are some additional considerations for when you're ready to meet threesome partners.

Bigger clubs and venues will have an online presence, and you should be able to find them by googling "sex club + my city," or "swinger club + my city." Be ready for the term "lifestyle" club, sometimes used as code for swinger. There may also be kink and BDSM spaces that have some parties that are more sex focused. Check out Fetlife.com for event listings as well as Meetup.com for sex-positive groups in your area. Some of these venues will even have a presence on other social media, like Facebook, Instagram, and Twitter.

Even before you attend one of these events, the social media pages for the venues or parties can be a good way to meet people who are open-minded and interested in multiperson play. Read the threads and comments for a while before you post to get an idea of the tone of the group and to see if personal-ad style posts are allowed or common.

Each event will have its own set of rules and its own culture, so be sure to read all of the posted event rules and any advice posts specific to the party or club. Then, when you go, try to have low expectations. A first visit is just a fact-finding mission. You're discovering if you like the vibe of the space and if the people seem like your kind of folks.

Many parties will have a host or hosts who you can chat with about what to expect, or who can possibly give you a tour of the space. Take advantage of these offers when they're available, because getting comfortable in the space will benefit you in the long run.

Some parties might be very pickup play oriented, and at others people will largely play with their dates or with people they had advance plans with. Either way, they can be a good opportunity to meet people.

Just because you meet someone at a club or party doesn't necessarily mean you have to play there. The benefit of playing in the space is built-in safety—being in public, and not having to share addresses. But the downsides can be that play is time limited, and it can be trickier to negotiate at a party that's loud and crowded. You may decide to exchange info and meet up another time, either for a date to get to know each other better, or to simply have the threesome in one of your homes.

If you are going to negotiate a first-time threesome at a party, be sure you've got any preexisting negotiations with your partner(s) down solid and that you know exactly what questions you want to ask the new person—and what answers you want to hear.

If threesomes and/or group play become a regular thing for you, parties can be a great space for that. Once you're comfortable with the setting and with the process of negotiation, it's helpful to have a neutral space to go. It can feel safer to not share addresses, and it can also feel more emotionally tidy to not bring new partners home.

Cruises and Retreats

While more on the swinger side of things, there are even cruises and resort takeovers for people in the "lifestyle."

If you're committed to your group sex fantasies and you've got time and money to spare, these events can be a way to have a sexual adventure and work on your tan all at the same time.

Private Parties

If you can't find what you're looking for, make it yourself!

While probably not a move for the absolute beginner, once you start to make sex-positive friends, hosting your own sexy party can be a great way to meet people for threesomes. And if you're feeling especially brave, you can even try hosting a (mildly) sexy party for a group of friends who aren't quite sure about this kind of thing yet.

There are many ways to have a sexy party—and they don't need to involve sex! In fact, it's helpful if at least your first one doesn't. As you're getting used to sex-positive spaces, and your friends are getting used to exploration, it's helpful to use a format people are familiar with and boundaries that only nudge at people's comfort zones. An old-fashioned make-out party is a great way to start. Spin the bottle isn't just for teenagers! It can be a wonderful icebreaker for exploration.

I suggest a few modern, consent-focused updates to the classic format. First, it's helpful if everyone in the room is willing to engage with everyone else. That doesn't have to mean kissing. The second suggestion is thinking outside the box for what each spin means. What about hugging or doing a little dance together? Maybe a piggyback ride or feeding each other something from the snack table. Get creative! And third, no one is ever pushed into anything. The person who spins proposes an activity, and the person who was spun on can accept that proposal or suggest something else. Keep going until you find something both people are comfortable with.

When inviting friends, let people know what they're in for. Explain what kind of party it is and what your reasons are for throwing it. These parties aren't necessarily about cruising your friends for possible threesome buddies, they're for cultivating a different kind of community. One in which people can explore and talk about their fantasies. From that kind of environment, all kinds of new experiences are possible—not just threesomes.

If kissing feels like too much, you can also throw a porn movie night—these work best with an older classic, something from the 1970s that's a bit lighthearted and also a bit more tame than modern fare.

You can also throw an erotica reading party, where everyone brings a sexy story to read aloud to the group. It can be something they've written, if they're feeling creative, or something from a book. People take turns reading, usually not more than four to eight minutes per person. And it's okay if some people just come to watch, as long as there are enough people taking turns to keep the evening going.

While these options might seem silly, they serve a purpose. They get your friends comfortable in sexually charged environments and make it feel safer to talk about sex—an opportunity we rarely get.

A quick walk through your local sex toy store or a search online will also bring up numerous sexy party games. Try card games or sexy versions of classics like Pictionary or Twister. Just having a group of friends talk about sexy topics, or share their own stories, can be a powerful experience.

Even if you never want to have threesomes or group sex, tamer sexy parties can be a great way to get a bit of a spark going, try something new, and expand your views around sexual expression.

Classes

If you live in a mid- to large-sized city, you almost certainly have venues offering classes on a variety of sexy topics. Depending on the venue and the class, sometimes there is a social or mixer aspect to the event. These classes draw people who are at least curious about sexy topics, and they can be a good place to make friends and build community—though they are not a place for cruising for hookups.

The added benefit is because it's a class, you're bound to learn something. So the outing should be worthwhile even if you don't strike up conversations with anyone.

Attending classes can also be a great way to start tiptoeing into sexy spaces with a partner or friend you're hoping to have threesomes with. While starting these conversations out of the blue might feel difficult, having the context of a class gives you an outline for the conversation. Try talking about the content of the class. How did it make you feel? What did you learn? Is there anything you disagreed with?

When you're looking for classes or deciding which is the right fit for you, pay attention to where the class is being held. Classes on sex, kink, and relationship topics can be held in venues ranging from sex toy stores to yoga studios to dungeons. Make sure you know what the space is so you can decide if it's some-where you'll feel comfortable.

Another benefit of classes is that they give you an "excuse" to be in a space. For example, if there's a class held in a dungeon or sex club, it's a great way to check out the venue in a nonplay setting. And that can make it feel easier to come back another time, because you'll know what you're getting into.

Polyamory Meet-ups

Many areas have meet-ups for polyamorous folks and other open relationship configurations. But this recommendation comes with reservations.

Because polyamory means engaging in multiple, ongoing, loving relationships, you should know that the polyamorous crowd will be especially sensitive to anything that seems like unicorn hunting. Be sure you're ready to follow the culture and etiquette of the group if you attend.

Meet-ups of this kind won't be for cruising for partners; rather they're a chance to get to know people who practice various forms of nonmonogamy. And yes, down the line, some of those people can become play partners.

Folks who are veterans of various forms of nonmonogamy are a fantastic resource for many of the questions you might be having. They're used to talking about and dealing with everything from jealousy to scheduling headaches. And if you approach with an open mind, and no fixed agenda, you may be able to learn a lot.

Polyamorous communities are also a wonderful place to learn about the joys of compersion. This is the term used to describe the joy you feel at seeing a partner's joy. In the poly world, this often means feeling happy for a partner when they've had a good date, or when they've met someone new they're excited about. But threesomes can be a wonderful source of compersion, too.

In a threesome, you've got a chance to see your partner or new friends enjoying new people and new experiences right in front of you. You can watch them finding hot chemistry, receiving compliments, and indulging fantasies.

Compersion is sometimes described as the opposite of jealousy, but I think that's an oversimplification. That said, some of the same experiences can lead to either response. Think about it as an opportunity to make a choice; when you see a partner with someone else, how are you going to respond? While we can't choose our gut reactions, we can train ourselves over time to respond in new ways.

Think Outside the Box

When I have coaching clients who want help with dating, one of the main pieces of advice I give them is to do the things they enjoy doing, and meet people who also like those things.

Like rock climbing? Start hanging around the climbing gym. Enjoy knitting? Find a stitch 'n bitch group. Whatever your hobby is, there are people getting together to do it in groups.

You may also find some unlikely overlaps. Events like comic-cons and sci-fi conventions often have such a big overlap with alternative lifestyles that they'll host panels on relationship issues. It shouldn't be such a surprise, really. Plenty of classic fantasy and sci-fi novels feature open relationships or a range of sexualities and identities.

In fact, I was recently asked to speak at a sci-fi and fantasy convention and found myself a bit baffled. While I like the genres, they're not what I write. But then I saw the lineup of panels, and they were tackling everything from kink to open relationships to communication—plus some erotica readings after dark!

Don't fake it if those kinds of events aren't your cup of tea, but do take a look at the lineup for your local events—you might be surprised what you find.

But What Do You Say?

You've put yourself out there and you've met someone you'd like to have a threesome with. So what do you actually say to make it happen?

Remember that if you've met someone in the wild, there are more variables than meeting someone online. Unless you've met someone in a space that's explicitly about sex or hookups, you have no idea if they're available. And even in a sexy space, there's no guarantee they'll be into you. So your approach needs to be friendly and polite.

When you strike up a conversation, make it about a shared interest—maybe about the event or activity you're partaking in. Ask the person about themselves. It's okay to flirt, but don't be overbearing. Keep body language in mind, too. Make sure you're not trapping someone in a corner or against a wall. If you see their eyes darting around the room, it's probably a good time to take a step back.

Make sure the person you're talking to knows if you're part of a couple. You don't want to get their hopes up for a one-on-one fling if that's not on the table. And if you're in a space where you feel comfortable, try to work into the conversation that you and your partner are in an open relationship, or open to multi-person play.

If you're in a space where cruising is welcome, try saying something like, "We both think you're super hot," or "You two are really sexy together," depending whether you're coming at this solo or partnered.

People like compliments, and being flattered, so that can be a good start as long as it's honest! Don't claim attraction where there isn't any. If you're really just into one of the people, don't bring the other along for the ride. And if half of your couple isn't game, don't force it.

What else could you say?

- "I/we have been fantasizing about having a threesome—is that something you might be into?"
- "Have you ever had a threesome before?"
- "I've been super curious about kissing two people at once."

It may take some practice if you haven't been on the market for a while. But you'll get the hang of it! Just remember that the very first conversation you have is unlikely to lead to a threesome. And, in fact, it might take quite a few approaches before something works out.

Don't let your frustration (or desperation) show. That'll be an instant turn-off to anyone you're talking to. So if you're feeling burned out, it's time to take a break and come back to it when you can have a positive outlook and approach.

12

THREESOME INTERLUDE

Parallel Play

There are a number of ways a parallel or *V*-shaped threesome can play out. Here's one example.

My friend Grace had a recent breakup and was starting to get out and socialize again. We went out for drinks, and she joked about needing to get laid. I started running though my mental rolodex of friends I could set her up with, and my friend Reid was at the top of the list. I mentioned him to her, but things didn't go further than that.

A couple weeks later, she and I went to a show together and Reid was one of the performers. As soon as he stepped on stage, she leaned over to whisper that he was exactly her type. A plan began to form in my mind.

Although Grace and I had fooled around a couple of times at parties, we were primarily platonic friends. Still, being party veterans, I knew we both had a solid understanding of how to navigate sexy spaces.

When the show was over, I told Grace that Reid was the

friend I'd told her about over drinks, and asked if she'd like to meet him. With a bit of a blush, she said yes.

We went to chat with him, and they were flirting right away. It was good to see her exploring this part of herself again. As he moved on to chat with other audience members, she and I checked in. Deciding there was no time like the present, we resolved to propose a threesome for that night.

While she and I weren't planning much in the way of direct play, having it be a group adventure would help keep things light and playful, and would create a nice buffer as they got to know each other and she got her feet wet with sex and dating again.

Reid had already been an occasional play partner of mine, and I'd been in threesomes and other group sex adventures with him in the past. Knowing him to be a direct person (and generally game for an adventure) I simply walked up to him and asked if he'd like to have a threesome with us that night. (While being that direct won't work in a lot of circumstances, it can be the right fit when you've cultivated a group of friends who regularly engage in these activities.) He feigned a bit of shyness but quickly agreed, and we made a plan to meet at his place.

Reid's house features a hot tub, which is a fantastic icebreaker for sexy times. The hot tub is a great excuse to get naked, but then just relax and chat as you ease into the situation. As we soaked, we eventually started a bit of negotiation. We checked in about boundaries as well as likes and dislikes. Although I was already familiar with Grace and Reid, they were just getting to know each other.

We moved to the bedroom, and she and I lay side by side, while Reid took turns kissing each of us. Luckily Grace and I both like to watch, so rather than being bored when we weren't the ones being kissed, we were getting just as much of a thrill from the voyeurism. And while I'd played with both of them before, there were no established couples in the bed, so everyone was coming together on fairly equal footing.

Next, Reid went down on me while Grace watched and stroked my body a bit. When he came up for air, he asked Grace how she felt about getting my fluids on her mouth—and she said she didn't want any fluid exchange. So Reid went to the bathroom to wash his face and rinse his mouth out.[5] When he came back, they kissed for a while and then he went down on her.

Since she and I weren't really playing, I was now free to reposition and engage some other way . . . and the position Reid was in allowed me plenty of access from the rear.

After a check-in, I grabbed a toy and some lube from his stash and began penetrating him from behind while he went down on her. This line-up of bodies was a hot way to play, with everyone's movements impacting each other even if not everyone was directly involved. As I thrust into him, it pushed his face further into her, and if she pressed up against him, it pushed him back into me.

With Reid in the middle, he got to receive a lot of stimulation—with his face between her legs and me inside him from behind. And Grace and I both had excellent views of everything going on, so in addition to the fun we were having with our own activities, we also had a personal sex show happening right in front of us.

Having things to watch, and listen to, can heighten the sexual experience and add to the overall feeling of high stimulation, even if you're not doing a ton of touching or receiving touch.

It can also mean extra stimulation when it comes to post-sex cuddles! When we were done playing, we were able to collapse into a pile together to snuggle and talk about the experience, which was a lovely way to end our evening together.

---

5 Read more about mouthwash in the safer-sex section.

ONLINE DATING/APP OPTIONS

Which Sites or Apps to Use

The world of online dating moves too quickly to have an exhaustive or accurate list of apps and websites in print, but check the resources section in the back of this book for places to start. More important is what to look for in an app and how to use it once you get set up.

With the increasing acceptance of polyamory and other open relationship styles, dating apps and sites have become more accommodating in order to remain relevant. OKCupid added features that allow you to not only say if you're already in a relationship, but to link to your partner's profile. And apps like Feeld came about specifically to help facilitate threesomes.

When deciding which app is right for finding threesomes, look for options that make it friendly for couples to use. Either an explicit option for a couples' profile or linking options, as mentioned above. That way, whichever side of the equation you're on, you'll be able to find the kind of people you're looking for.

The other thing that's important is making sure there are

enough people in your area on the app to make it relevant. A brand new app with stellar options won't get you very far if only a couple dozen people in your city are using it—unless you get very lucky! Apps like Tinder are so widely adopted they can be worth checking out, even though (as of this writing) they don't have explicit couples' options.

Whichever app you decide to use, be sure you're playing by their rules. For example, a site specially aimed at women looking for women wouldn't be a good place for a heterosexual couple to make a profile.

Read some reviews online and see what people are saying about each app. Aside from different rules and tools, they're likely to have different cultures and activity levels.

Beyond dating apps, there are also a variety of websites you might find useful. Some explicitly allow personal-ad type content, and others don't—not every useful website is geared towards dating. Some are more community or event focused, but they can still be a great way to meet people. Websites like FetLife or Kasidie function as social media more than dating apps, but can be useful not only for the connections they facilitate, but because you may learn about your local scene, culture, or events.

On some sites explicit photos and text will be removed, and your account may even be suspended or banned. So if you're hoping for x-rated content, that's a factor that will drive your website choice. If you want to go all-in with naked pictures, websites like FetLife might be your best bet.

Don't disqualify other social media—even Facebook can be a useful tool! There are subgroups for everything, and if you spend time in open relationship groups, you may meet potential partners there.

Keep in mind on social networks that explicit cruising will

likely get you booted out. So take a while to learn the tone of the group and to just get to know people.

Profile Pictures

Dating apps these days are very photo focused. In fact, some people let their photos do all the talking and don't include any profile text at all. While I wouldn't suggest that approach, it's true that your photos are an essential element to get right. You're not just showing what you look like, you're showing who you are.

With most of the apps being largely photo and swipe based, your pictures really need to do a lot of the heavy lifting for you. Find pictures to share that show something about your personality. Being cute certainly helps, but being interesting goes a long way too.

Share pictures of you engaging in a favorite activity, whether that's rock climbing or reading. Share pictures snuggling with your pets or playing an instrument. Whatever you choose, make sure it's a real thing about you, not just a dating app photo opp.

You want your photos to not only grab people's attention but to be a conversation starter. "Oh, you like that book? Me too!" The more potential ways to connect to other people, the better.

Let's break that down a little further.

Most apps allow anywhere from five to ten pictures. And while you don't need to use every slot, you should have a minimum of three pictures (more if there are two of you).

Here are some categories to consider: a great picture of your face (maybe headshot style), a full body shot, an activity or personality photo, a photo with a pet, and a dressed up photo.

A group shot can be okay if your friends consent to being used on a dating app, and as long as it isn't your main (or only) photo. No one is willing to do the work to figure out which person in the group you are.

While the selfie is ubiquitous these days, try not to have

exclusively selfies on your profile. And if you do have selfies, make sure they're good ones. Be mindful of your background. Don't take pictures in the bathroom or with a pile of dirty laundry behind you, or in full view of your unmade bed. Aim for clean and cozy environments or nice, bright, outdoor spaces.

Remember that selfie technology has advanced! You're not limited to holding your phone out in your hand at an awkward angle and hoping for the best. Consider getting a cheap tripod or propping your phone on something and using the timer function. This will allow you to get more of your body in the shot as well as experiment with better angles.

We also have a lot of photo editing software at our disposal, and there are plenty of apps that do most of the work for you, so you don't need any photoshop skills. Consider blurring the background a bit or using portrait mode to keep you as the center of attention. You can also make the photo a little brighter or more crisp.

Do remember that people are photo filter savvy, and if your photo is edited beyond recognition, it'll show. A little adjusting is fine, but you should still look like yourself—wrinkles, freckles, and all.

You want to avoid cliché while still including images that show your personality. So, while I'd avoid pics of you with a tiger cub, my profile, for example, does have a picture of me in the Paris Catacombs, which gives helpful insight into my personality.

Ideally you'll have a mix of selfies and photos taken of you by other people. It should be an easy ask of a friend, and you can even trade places, getting pics of each other.

A professional photographer is also a great option. Photography has moved well beyond the glamour shot, and it's not difficult to find a photographer who is familiar with taking headshots or personality pics. Often you can get a combination of both.

What about sexy photos? This will largely come down to your personality and the rules of the site you're on. Some dating apps will pull photos they consider too racy, while some websites allow full nudity and even sex acts in the photos (or videos!).

If you're going the professional photography route, you might even want to do some boudoir shots. These can be great solo or with a partner, and it's worthwhile to have a professional to help you figure out your angles.

Just remember that showing a lot of skin in your photos will give the impression that you're looking primarily for casual sex. If that's true for you—great! If not, consider keeping your clothes on for now, and sending sexy pictures later on if messaging goes in that direction.

Profile Language

Thanks to the internet, it's easier than ever to find other people who share your interests. But there's also a lot of information to slog through. And since you won't have someone's attention for long, it's important to get the essentials out in a concise and eye-catching way.

Your profile should reflect information about who you are. That means, who you *really* are. Faking it isn't only unethical, it just doesn't work. You need to find people who are into you, and excited about your interests. And they're out there. You just need some patience to find them.

For starters, share some interesting facts about yourself—fun things that another person could connect with, and enough information that someone can get a sense of your personality. If it's a couples' profile, have a paragraph about each of you and something about the relationship. Maybe talk about how you met, or activities you enjoy doing together. Let people get a sense of what you're like as a couple.

After you've talked about yourself, make it clear what you're looking for. If you're on the app specifically for threesomes, say so. You don't want to waste the time of people who are only looking for one-on-one dating.

Don't make it all about sex. Even if that's the primary thing you want to do, you'll still need to get along as people. If you can't at least have a conversation, it's going to be tricky to have sex. So have enough things in common that if you met at a cocktail party, you could happily chat for thirty minutes or more.

Don't go negative. That means about yourself or others. No self-deprecating humor here. Don't apologize for your photos or for a profile that's still in progress. Instead, don't put anything out there you don't feel good about!

Don't list things you don't want—instead, say what you do want. Consider each sentence and find a way to frame it in a positive way. What about if you're frustrated with the partner search? It's okay to feel that way—but make sure it doesn't show in your profile (or your messages). Being negative is a big turn-off, and if you're trashing online dating, you're also trashing anyone who is reading your profile.

Maybe you don't want friends or colleagues to know that you're looking for dates or threesome buddies—what then? It's certainly a real concern that you could run into people you know on a dating app. So spend some time considering whether that's a problem for you.

While you can have a more anonymous profile that doesn't include face pictures, or pictures you can be identified by, that's also going to make your partner search more difficult. Being unwilling to show your face can read as a red flag to people, even if you've got a good reason. So if you're going the privacy route, try to explain why. For example, "I work with kids so no face pictures here, but I'm happy to send pics after we match."

★ ★ ★

If you're on the kind of site that's explicit enough to say what you're looking for sexually, make sure you're also saying what you have to offer.

For example, "Looking to fulfill my partner's fantasy," looks not only like half the couple might not be into it, but like the third's pleasure doesn't come into the equation. How about saying you love to cook nice meals and give massages?

To sum up: a profile should say who you are as a person, not just sexually. You should be ready to connect with people as people, on multiple levels. And you should be giving as much as you're hoping to get.

Couples' Profile Logistics

If you're creating a profile as a couple, you'll want to make sure that both of you approve of the pictures used and any profile text, too. This can be a great time to look through pictures of the two of you together and remember all the fun you've already had on your own!

Ideally the main picture on your couples' profile will be of the two of you together. You want the fact that it's a couple's profile to be as transparent as possible, because people won't take kindly to being surprised with that information after they've gotten their hopes up about just one of you.

What about the logistics of swiping? Is the online hunt something you'll only do when you're together, or is one person leading the charge? Either way, be sure to negotiate how that will go.

While the idea of doing it all together sounds nice, that also means dedicating a chunk of your shared time to the process—so it may depend on how much time you've got to spare. If one of you has more free time, or is more savvy with online dating, it could make sense for them to do a lot of the advance work, and only check in when there are decisions to be made.

Keep in mind that if one of you is doing all the swiping and chatting, that can lead to an imbalance that can cause jealousy. You may decide that in the name of fairness you should each create a couples' profile of your own, so you can each swipe on your own time.

While some sites let you have an actual couple's profile, many others require work-arounds. That means you may have to choose one gender option for your profile. In addition to having couples' options, some sites have finally offered a broader range of gender choices, while some are still limited to male and female. Which is all to say, if you and your partner aren't the same gender, you'll have to pick one to represent you on the app.

You may have to conduct your own social experiment to see what works best. Online dating anecdotes make contradictory arguments. I've heard some say that having a profile marked as female will lead to matches with a lot of queer women and nonbinary folks who may want nothing to do with men or couples. But this experience is far from universal.

Luckily, if you each make your own profile, you can test these hypotheses on your own. Or, if you have one profile, you can always delete and start over if you're not getting the results you're looking for.

Simply scrolling through the apps together and looking at potential matches can be a big part of the fun. What conversations do other people's profiles bring up? Does seeing other people's images get you excited about the prospect of playing together, or are you getting a knot of nerves in your stomach? Remember that how you feel during the partner search is a good indication about how you're feeling about the whole idea.

Word Choice

Dating profiles are getting shorter and shorter, which makes word choice all the more important. You need to make clear who you are and what you're looking for in as little space as possible. That means it's doubly important to consider what message the words and phrases you're choosing will send.

Whether solo dating or looking for threesomes, you'll find the phrase "no drama" across online platforms. All too often this translates into, "don't have any needs that will inconvenience me."

Listen, we all want to be dating mature adults with solid life skills, and you're going to be screening for things like emotional maturity and communication skills as you read profiles and exchange first messages. So don't get things off on the wrong foot with turn-off phrases like this.

In fact, avoid negatives all together. Instead of saying what you don't want, speak in positive terms and articulate what you do want.

Another phrase you'll see is *DDF* or *drug and disease free*. On its surface, that might sound reasonable, but there are connotations hiding beneath the surface. For one, we're no longer associating the word 'disease' with things associated with sex. That's why the term STI has replaced STD. Another problem with this term is the close association between drugs and disease. There's no reason to assume that people who use drugs have STIs, or that people with an STI use drugs.

The DDF term is also misleading and potentially obsolete because the people using it are rarely considering alcohol or marijuana under the category of drugs. In fact, you're likely to see the term *420 friendly* in the very same posts. Any substance use should be specifically discussed as a safety and consent matter, but the language used shouldn't reinforce stigma.

Another unfortunate word you'll see when people are discussing STI status is "clean." In fact, this one is pretty common.

The problem is that saying clean implies that the opposite is dirty—and that framing further shames and stigmatizes STIs, which leads more people to be unwilling to have the conversation, or unwilling to disclose their status. Plenty of people live with STIs like HIV or HSV and that doesn't disqualify them as sex partners. It's simply a conversation to be had. So make sure you're not contributing to sex-negative stigma around STIs with your word choice.

Have you ever noticed how the world tends to rally together in shared hatred of certain words? *Moist* comes to mind as universally hated. (I don't mind it, but maybe I'm just contrary.) One word that gets people's hackles up, and is therefore best to avoid in your profiles or personal ads, is *female*. This isn't to say that you can't post that you're interested in women, but few things get people as riled up as using the term *females* to refer to women. In fact, there are articles across the web, from Jezebel[xi] to Buzzfeed,[xii] urging people not to use this word. Similarly, the word *ladies* can cause the same nails-on-chalkboard cringe for a lot of people, so you're better off avoiding it.

Likewise, avoid mentioning what body types or physical attributes you're looking for in a partner. You're not ordering a RealDoll. And while everyone has their own preferences, you can screen for attraction without advertising that you only want to talk to people with the measurements of a runway model.

In fact, avoid all objectifying language—and that's not just about bodies. Don't say anything that makes the third sound like an object or sex toy. For example, saying you're looking for a birthday or anniversary present for your partner—that sounds like a thing, not a person.

And as an aside, if you are hoping for a threesome to celebrate a special occasion, remember that you're setting up a high-stakes scenario that's at risk of backfiring. Especially for a first threesome, it's best to try it without a particular timeline in mind. Have a nice dinner for your special occasion, then have a three-some for the hell of it.

One last word that might give people the wrong idea—the word *discreet* gets thrown around by people who are keeping secrets or cheating on a partner, so its use might raise red flags. If you're aiming for some amount of privacy, that's fine, but consider how you express that information.

First Messages and Beyond

First messages should be friendly, not explicit. A quick scroll through my own Tinder shows that the last couple who picked me up started by asking what book I'd read most recently. And it was a full week of chit chat before I asked them what they were looking for. And the answer? Not just potential sex partners, but friends.

Making friends as an adult can be difficult, so why waste the opportunity? If you like someone enough to have sex with them, there's a good chance they're friend material too. They're also likely open-minded and sex-positive. Making friends on dating apps, whether you also have sex with them or not, can be a great way to start building new community.

When messaging from a couple's profile, make it clear who is doing the writing. Is one half of the partnership doing most of the outreach? This can be as simple as signing your message with the name of who's writing. Or if every message is a joint effort, say that too. People want to know who they're talking to.

That same couple who picked me up with book talk? All the writing was done by the woman. And when we exchanged numbers, it was her number she gave me. Even after roughly a year of chatting and occasional threesome dates, I've only spoken directly to her on the app or by text.

As much as I wish everything were gender neutral, I have found that when an MF couple is picking up another F, it can often work best if the women talk first, or do some of the first flirting. That tends to be where the mismatch or discomfort is going to be, if there's going to be any. So making sure the women get along and are into each other is a good step to making sure things go smoothly overall.

No matter how many messages you're writing, don't copy and paste the same first message to everyone. Savvy online daters can smell generic from a mile away. Make sure you actually read the profiles of the people you're interested in, look at their pictures, and craft a message that's actually for and about them.

Do you have hobbies in common? Do they have a cute pet? Do you have similar taste in movies, music, or books? Remember, the conversation doesn't have to be about sex right off the bat—start by building rapport.

Also on the no-no list: unsolicited explicit photos. Don't send pictures of nudity or sex acts unless the conversation has already gotten sexy and you've gotten clear permission to send them. This should go without saying, but anatomy-textbook worthy photos of genitals don't get you dates.

If you're going to be messaging for a while, you've got logistical choices to make. It can be helpful to move to text or to a messaging app that can easily manage a three-way chat.

Messaging styles differ. Some people like to message for a while, maybe even weeks, before meeting up. Others like to meet sooner rather than later, to find out if there's chemistry before investing too much time. You may find it helpful to have a phone call or video chat so all three people can get a feeling for each other. This is more efficient than messaging and less of an investment than a date.

Don't be pushy. Take no for an answer. And remember that sometimes silence is your answer. If you don't get an answer to your message, feel free to send one friendly check-in. But if you don't hear back after two messages, let it go.

Always be sure that you're representing yourself accurately. A single person shouldn't be using the lure of a threesome to get a date, posing as a couple. And a couple shouldn't pose as a unicorn to arrange a voyeur or cuckold scenario. Stick with the classic rule and treat other people the way you'd like to be treated.

When you're trying to get to more explicit planning in your conversation, try questions like, "What are you looking for?" Not only is this a great way to segue into threesome talk, but it's also a way to show you care about the other person's interests.

Here's what one woman had to say about messaging someone they met online:

Our first threesome experience went really well. My then partner and I had been dating about six months. I'm a queer woman, he identifies as heteroflexible. We met Alice online and she and I texted a lot during the day. I made a group chat for us because it was more fun to include all three parties.

All the chatting was helpful for the two of us to feel comfortable and to have an idea of what we wanted. By the time we were in bed together, I knew how she liked to be touched and some of her turn-ons. One thing that I loved about this particular encounter was hearing the two of them talk about how to get me off. He was showing her what I like, and the combination of their efforts was pretty fabulous.

One thing I would do differently in the future is share more about how my partner and I interact. There were a few moments when I had to stop to tell her that I was ok with things like deep throating and having my hair pulled.

> *She was fine once she knew I was consenting, but it would have been better to disclose that ahead of time. We planned to meet up again, but she found a monogamous partner the next month.*

Send Nudes?

The idea of sexting is pretty ubiquitous these days. And sharing sexy messages can be a lot of fun, whether with an existing partner or someone you're thinking of meeting up with. If you're considering some sexy chat, there are a few things to think about.

While there are some apps that make messaging and sending photos a bit more secure, always consider anything that you put on the internet or in text to be a thing that is now out of your control, and potentially shareable. Even in the case of "secure" apps, or apps that delete your photos within a certain timeframe, screenshots can still be taken. While you might not be running for political office or making yourself a blackmail target—how would you feel if you saw your photo posted somewhere without your permission?[6] And while that might not be a likely outcome, it's safest not to post or send anything you wouldn't want the world to see.

If you decide to go for it, have fun with the process! Taking sexy pictures of yourself can be empowering. Find clothes you feel good in, figure out some good lighting, and consider your background.

All of the tips from the profile photo section apply here, plus a few more. For starters, even if you're not worried about privacy, decide if you want your face in the picture. You can send body

---

6   Luckily the law is starting to catch up with technology, and in some cases it's now illegal to share photos or videos without permission—what is sometimes called *revenge porn*. Also worth noting, it is always illegal to share pictures of minors—even of yourself! There have been prosecutions even of teens sending pictures to each other.

shots that don't include your face, recognizable tattoos, etc., if that feels safer.

Consider embracing the art of the tease. Just because you're going to share dirty pictures doesn't mean you need to give everything away. It can be sexy to leave something to the imagination and leave your recipient wanting more. Try pictures with lingerie or underwear on, or tight clothes that give a hint of what's beneath. Play with simply pulling a shirt up or down, giving an extra hint of skin. You can also use lighting to your advantage here, deciding which parts stay in the shadows.

Sending sexy pictures can be a fun way to build anticipation and even to start talking about what things you might want to do together. Just make sure no one gets left out. It can help if you start some kind of group chat so everyone can be included. Or, if one person is driving the texting on behalf of someone else, making it clear if the pictures are being shared.

Essential sexting etiquette: always ask first! Don't surprise someone with an explicit picture. Make sure it's something they're interested in receiving and also that it's a good time. You never know who might be able to see someone's phone screen, and you don't want to create an awkward situation with someone's boss or kids, for example.

And if you've been blessed with a (consensual) sexy photo, be sure to say thank you and to shower the person with compliments. Sending pictures can be vulnerable, so make sure the other person feels good about sharing with you.

Have Patience and a Thick Skin

Everyone will tell you that online dating can be kind of a slog. The same things that make it useful—like having so many people available—can also be a downside. With the next swipe always just around the corner, some people don't put a whole lot of effort into any particular match.

Dating books and articles will all show you some depressing statistics. The likelihood of making a match is low, as is receiving a response to a message. But believe it or not, that has a silver lining. It means it's not about you! Online dating is hard for everyone, so if you're not getting the results you're looking for, it doesn't mean you're a bad match, it can just mean that online dating is a tricky numbers game.

It's still a good idea to optimize your chances by working on your photos, profile, and messaging game, but if you're doing your best then what's needed is patience.

You're going to "like" people who don't like you back. You're going to send messages that go unanswered. You're going to start conversations that end up going cold for no apparent reason. You may even start talking to someone you realize later is a bot or fake profile.

Go into this adventure with a thick skin and a sense of humor. You'll need to be able to brush off these misses and move on to what's next. If you start to feel overwhelmed or discouraged, it's time to take a break. Remember that this is supposed to be fun, and if it stops being fun, what's the point?

If you've been with it for a while and you're just not getting the results you want, take a break and take stock. Is there something about your approach that needs work or could be improved? Are you in a small enough town that pickings are slim? Is there something about the online format that makes it so you can't put your best foot forward?

Before giving up, try tweaking all the variables. Change out pictures, change your profile or bio, and change your messaging strategy. If online dating is still a bust, try focusing on some of the in-person options for meeting people.

NEGOTIATION

Expectations, Boundaries, and Limits

What are you hoping to get from this threesome? Is there a particular fantasy you have in mind? A kind of experience you're hoping to have? It's helpful to lay all of this out during negotiations so that everyone involved can help make your fantasies happen, or make clear that they want something else up front. It's difficult to get your needs met if you don't articulate what they are. So you need to be honest with yourself, and then open and honest with the other people involved.

If there are boundaries or limits, all parties need to know about them. Or if there are particular acts or positions that are off the table—again, make that clear. It will feel stilted and awkward in the moment if certain activities are being avoided or dodged without explanation, and it's all too easy for someone to cross a boundary if they don't know it exists. Don't set someone up for failure by not informing them what everyone in the situation needs.

Remember, just because there's a boundary doesn't mean there aren't still a lot of fun options. For example, maybe there's an existing couple in the mix, and they only want penetration between them. As you'll see in the positions section, there are lots of ways to play with multiple people beyond penetration—or by having some people involved in penetration and other people involved in oral sex.

Don't frame a boundary as something that limits your fun; think of it as something that will help you get more creative as you decide what to do.

Once a boundary has been set, consider it non-negotiable for that encounter. Arousal can have similar effects to intoxication, making it a bad idea to try to take things further than initially agreed upon. And it's not a good move to ask more than once after a boundary has been set or someone has said no—at worst it can even be coercive.

A few years ago, I was at a play party and ended up playing with a couple who had never played with a third before. Not only that, but the other woman was also inexperienced with women, so this encounter was a lot of firsts for her. During the play she asked for breaks a couple of times. She'd go get some water, or some air, and then come back when she was ready. Whenever she left the space, all play would stop. Eventually she was done for the night, having had an encounter that stayed above the waist all around.

Whether he wasn't paying attention or simply wasn't inter-ested in his partner's limits, the male half of the couple tried to keep things going, and I had to firmly remind him that his partner had called a stop to the encounter.

Behavior like that is a good way to make sure that someone won't play with you again—and maybe that your partner won't feel safe exploring with you again, either. When a boundary has been stated, it's everyone's job to remember and respect it.

Avoiding "Rules"

What's the difference between a rule and a boundary? One way to think about this issue is that boundaries are about you, and rules are about other people. Are you setting a boundary to protect yourself, or making a rule to control other people? An example of this might be saying that during a threesome, you don't want to be kissed on the mouth. You've set a boundary that you're not comfortable with kissing in this encounter. What could make it a rule is saying the other two people in the threesome aren't allowed to kiss.

It's largely semantic. Some boundaries may still be problematic, and some rules may be fine. What's essential is that you have a say in the negotiation of any agreements you're going to be a part of. It's also helpful if all the agreements apply equally to everyone involved. In the example above, the person who doesn't want to be kissed could propose that there's no kissing at all in the threesome. So, while this could be called a rule because it controls other people's behavior, you're also being given the opportunity to agree or not, and it will apply to everyone equally. (Versus the existing couple kissing each other in front of you, while you're not allowed to kiss one or both of them.)

So, is something being framed as telling you what you can do? Or is the couple saying, "Let's all do this together?"

It's always helpful to frame things in a positive light. Using the kissing example, let's say you're tempted to ask the other two people in the threesome not to kiss each other (basically setting a rule)—before doing so, pause and ask yourself why you want that. If it's because of a fear of jealousy or of being left out, what's a way you can address that by adding something to the encounter, rather than taking something away?

Instead of saying the other two people can't kiss, could you meet the same needs by letting them know you're feeling sensitive about being left out, and would like a lot of attention paid to you? Could you say that you really like to receive a lot of kissing and touching and attention? Spend some time thinking about both of those options see how they feel.

Now think about how hearing each of those requests would feel to the other people involved.

Asking people not to kiss each other is limiting what other people can do and controlling their behavior. And if kissing is something that comes naturally to them during a sexual encounter, they're going to have to keep catching themselves when they have the impulse to kiss—which could end up being a serious distraction during play. Overall, this could have a big impact on their level of enjoyment.

Now imagine how it would feel for them to know you're feeling a little sensitive and would like to receive a lot of attention. Remembering to do something is easier than remembering not to. Every time they glance in your direction, or any time there's a shift in position, they can make sure to include you or to give you some extra kissing or touching. Framing this request in the positive allows them to add ideas to the mix, which makes for a much easier flow than trying to remove something.

There's also a different emotional reaction. Dictating controlling rules that someone has to follow can create some resentment in response. But being up front about feeling vulnerable and asking for something you need is more likely to receive compassion and empathy in response. Which of these feelings would you rather have in your threesome?

This doesn't mean setting limits is a bad idea. You need to have limits. It's important to take care of yourself and feel empowered to say no when you need to. Just think carefully about what your boundaries are, and if the limit you're setting is actually going to get you the outcome you're looking for.

★ ★ ★

Remember, too, that every rule we set is a place where something can go wrong. If you end up setting arbitrary rules that aren't really that important, you're also setting a lot of landmines and potential opportunities for feelings to get hurt. Each rule is a place where there can be a misunderstanding or where something can be forgotten. So make sure that whatever agreements are set in place are both necessary and well understood by everyone involved.

Turn-Ons and Turn-Offs

Especially if it's been a while since you had sex with someone new, you might be taking it for granted that a partner knows what you like and don't like. But with someone new, you'll have to teach them. (And existing partners can probably use a refresher, too.)

When we're negotiating sex or play, we usually list the activities or toys that are on the table and those that are off limits. But don't forget to talk about the rest of the experience. Not just what you want to *do*, but how you want to *feel*.

Are you looking for an experience that's rough and tumble, or sweet and sensual? Do you want to feel cherished and cared for, or wildly desired? All of these feelings and more are possible, and if you think about the feelings, rather than just the activities, you'll give your play partners a lot more information to work with.

What about how you like to be touched? Do you like soft caresses or a firm grip? Are you ticklish? Extra sensitive anywhere on your body? Do you like a little bit of pain or intense sensation? How do you feel about fingernails raking across your skin?

What about the ways that you respond during sex? Is there anything unique or unexpected about the way you show pleasure or displeasure? Do you go nonverbal when you're about to have an orgasm? Try and think of anything a new partner should know before sex gets started.

Planning sex with a new person is a chance not only to explore brand new things, but to explore your own desires and interests all over again.

Logistics

Some people find threesomes daunting because of the actual logistics. And it's true, figuring out what's going to happen with three people can be a little trickier than with two. But with advance planning, there's no reason for the logistics to slow you down. Here are some questions for you to consider.

Where will the threesome happen? Is it at one of the participants' homes or somewhere neutral like a sex club or hotel?

On the most basic level, you need to make sure there's enough space. If someone's in a dorm room with only a twin bed, it's going to be difficult to roll around with three people—unless you're prepared to play on the floor. So the decision of where to go can sometimes be as simple as figuring out who has the biggest bed.

As for safety—how do you feel about giving out your address? There are safety considerations both for someone knowing where you live, and also for going to someone's home. If neither of these options feel good, but you still want to play, that's when a hotel room or public play space might be a good fit.

What about privacy? If some or all of the people involved don't live alone, it can be tricky to bring a partner home, let alone two. Have a conversation about options and what will make everyone the most comfortable.

Who's in charge of supplies? It's probably a good idea if everyone brings their favorite safer sex supplies, as well as sex toys. Having too much is never a problem, but you don't want to run out. And if there's something special you want for the event—like a strap-on harness—you might want to remind whoever owns the special thing to remember to bring it along.

How will timing work—when does it start, when does it end? Are there bedtimes to consider or early mornings at work?

If you're saying drinks at 9:00 p.m., realistically you're not getting to someone's home until 10 at the very earliest, then you're probably going to talk and flirt until at least 11, then you've got a couple hours for sex . . . and before you know it, it's time to get up for work the next morning.

If schedules allow, plan your threesome for when everyone has the next day off, or at least a late start. And see if you can get things started earlier in the evening. If you're a night owl maybe it's no problem, but consider that it can be a good three to four hours after meeting up before you get around to sex. And I, for one, am not at my best when it's past my bedtime.

It's also helpful to have a predefined end time for the three-some date. That can save you some of the awkwardness at the end of the night when it's time to leave, or when you want someone else to go. If you've agreed in advance, you can just say, "Oh, look at the time." Otherwise you might all be in a happy snuggle pile and then realize you need to start negotiating whether or not this is an overnight.

Speaking of overnights—are any of the people spending the night together? It's a good idea to decide in advance if there's an overnight happening. Not only will you need to pack the appropriate supplies, but you don't want to try and navigate this question in the middle of the night, when people might be tired or loopy from sex.

If your threesome is between people who are all involved

with each other to some degree, it's also useful to make clear if no one at all is spending the night together, or if two people are staying overnight and the third is going home. Whatever you decide, just make sure no one is surprised with this information when they're loopy and tired.

If you're not spending the night together, how will the evening come to a close? Hopefully you've set an end time, but are there any other ways you can end the evening on a high note? One couple I sleep with is in the habit of bringing over homemade desserts. So after sex we're motivated to get out of bed because there's pie, or chocolate mousse, or some other wonderful creation. Sharing a sweet treat is a great capstone for the night's activities, and also gives us a little closing ritual to smooth their transition out the door.

Does everyone have transportation? And will this be affected by potential intoxication? If you're not spending the night together, it's important to know how everyone is getting home. Are they counting on a bus or train that stops running at a certain time? Were they planning to drive but now they've had too much to drink? More than once I've ended up with an overnight guest because it got too late for them to leave. If that's not an acceptable outcome for you, make sure you've planned ahead.

Taking Breaks

When my mother first gave me the sex talk, I had one question: what if you have to go to the bathroom? Her answer was simple and to the point—you excuse yourself and go. What 10-year-old me didn't know to ask was: what if you need a bathroom break from a threesome?

That may sound like another silly question, but think about it. You get up to pee, come back into the room a couple minutes later, and the two people you left in bed are fully immersed in some activity, maybe not even looking up as you come back in. How does that make you feel?

Maybe it's no problem at all for you, and you simply dive back in. Or maybe you feel left out and can't imagine inserting yourself back into the activities. You might not know which of those camps you fall in until you're in that situation.

So it's a great idea to negotiate how bathroom breaks (or any other breaks) will work in advance. For beginner threesomes, it's the safest call to say the activities will pause anytime all participants aren't present and accounted for. Then when everyone is back in the room, or back in the bed, you can dive back into whatever was happening.

Aside from needing to pee, what about other breaks? It's important that anyone can call a time out at any time, for any reason. That's true for any kind of sex, and especially true for threesomes or group sex, when there are even more feelings and logistics to manage. And if someone does need a break, it's everyone else's job to be a good sport about it. It will be easiest to do this if you've discussed taking breaks when you're negotiating, before any clothes have come off. It can even be a good idea to take a few pre-planned breaks, just to make sure everyone has a chance to catch their breath and check in with themselves and each other.

If you start to feel overwhelmed, it's okay to ask for a pause. Check in with yourself, check in with the other people, and then decide if there are adjustments you can make that will make it comfortable to continue. Pushing yourself will only get you to a less happy breaking point later on.

What kind of adjustments can you make? Possibilities include scaling back in intensity, changing to a more familiar activity, or shifting the center of attention. If you've been trying a sex act that's brand new to you, how about shelving that and just kissing for a while? Or if you were in a supporting role and that stopped feeling good, what about asking the other two people to focus touch on you for a while?

Don't force yourself to continue—it's far better to call it a night and try again another time than to push yourself too far and have an experience you regret, which may leave a bad taste in your mouth about threesomes.

Power Dynamics

We'll talk about explicit kink power dynamics later on, but there are other forms of power and control—and they're not always negotiated. It's a good idea to think about the power dynamics of your threesome, even in a vanilla context.

Who is the driving force? Who is calling the shots? In a threesome it can be helpful if someone is confidently moving the action forward—as long as everyone is on board. If someone is helpfully leading the way, that's great. But if it feels like someone is pushing, or directing a less enthusiastic partner or partners, that can be a problem. Sometimes people have such a clear idea about the threesome of their dreams, they start playing choreographer in the moment. But that can spoil the fun for everyone.

When you're negotiating your threesome, have a conversation about this. Is someone more experienced or full of more ideas? Does everyone want to empower them to be a group leader? Maybe someone is better at the scheduling aspects and takes charge of arranging dates and times for get-togethers.

Are all power dynamics transparent and consensual? While it can be super hot to play with power, make sure any power dynamic at play has been negotiated and agreed to by all parties. If you sense a power imbalance among the people involved, that can complicate consent.

Does it seem like someone is just being dragged along? Does

someone appear to be calling the shots in a way not everyone agreed to? These should be big red flags.

Try to have these conversations first so you know what to expect, and if you notice power imbalances during your three-some that weren't discussed, feel free to speak up.

Intoxication

An awful lot of threesome stories start with people at a bar or at home drinking. You hear about drunken threesomes that people can't even remember the next day—and is that really what we want from a fantasy we've been looking forward to?

Aside from being a waste of an opportunity, substance use of any kind alters our perception, and should be taken into account when considering everybody's ability to make judgment calls or give consent.

It's understandable to want some liquid courage when you're going out on a limb and trying something new, but getting tipsy (or high) before your threesome adventure can backfire in a number of ways. On the purely practical side, alcohol has a number of side effects that can get in the way of your sexual performance. From erection difficulties to vaginal dryness, cocktails might not be your friend. And beyond your genitals, drinking can cause headaches as well as tiredness—none of which contribute to arousal.

Another risk is that lowering inhibitions with substances can mean that boundaries you decided on in advance get forgotten in the moment. Or that you dive into play without even having a conversation about boundaries. Being intoxicated can also bring out aspects of your personality that are less welcome in a three-some—everything from being pushier than usual to more shy or withdrawn.

If you feel that you need to be altered in order to have a threesome, it could be a sign that you're not ready for this adventure just yet—and that's okay! Better to go slow and do things you feel good about sober than to push yourself and regret something later.

Everyone has a different relationship to various substances, and if you are used to marijuana for medical purposes, for example, some level of altered state may be your normal. What's important is knowing what a baseline is for you—and your partners—so you don't run into any surprises in the moment.

Take into consideration whether this is your first threesome with a particular combination of people, or if you're all familiar with each other already. If you're all regular partners, you might feel comfortable being altered while having your tryst, because you have a better idea of everyone's needs and boundaries. But if anyone new is in the mix, you might not even know what their baseline looks like, which can make it tricky to judge how intoxicated someone even is.

Think I'm overstating the problems of intoxication? Here's an example from a friend of mine:

I had an impromptu threesome with a girlfriend and her coworker. They'd gone out to drinks and then come back to my house to hang out. They smoked some weed, one thing led to another, and then they were making out. After a bit they suggested we all fool around.

At the time, I didn't know better. I should have stopped to have some kind of discussion. Instead I just went for it, and we all went in the bedroom and had a good time. We cuddled a little afterwards, and then I took them both to their homes.

The next day, both of them were calling me and blaming me for roping them into something they didn't want to do.

> *Even though it was their idea, and they started making out with each other first, they were the ones drinking and smoking weed, so I became the bad guy.*
>
> *I know now that, had I stopped and had conversations with them and discussed boundaries, if nothing else, the fallout the next day would've been less.*

You have to ask yourself, is having a threesome worth the relationship and friendship fallout after the fact, if not everyone feels good about what happened? Not only that, but depending on what country or state you're in, there are laws on the books that cover whether someone is even capable of giving consent when they're intoxicated.

Remember, if something seems too good to be true, it probably is. Better to wait and see if people are still into the idea when everyone is sober. If so, you can always schedule to get together again.

Play Party Negotiation

Going to a play party means planning for being in a potentially loud and crowded space, where it may be difficult to check in on the fly. So it's helpful to negotiate in advance as much as you possibly can, to avoid trying to make snap decisions at the party.

For starters, decide why you're going. As with the options we've already covered, maybe you're going as a way to explore a sexual environment, or to meet a potential third. Knowing why you're going helps begin the discussion about what you're going to do there.

For example, if you're going to a party to explore the environment and watch people play, maybe one of the pre-negotiations is that you're not playing with any other people on that visit.

Maybe that sounds pretty simple, but think of it this way—

what happens if you don't discuss this in advance, and then at the party, someone approaches one or both of you? Suddenly you're on the spot in an environment that doesn't lend itself to lengthy, thoughtful conversations, and you've got a decision to make. All too often, this leads to trouble. Maybe both people are trying to guess what the other wants, and they guess wrong. It's common for people to not want to disappoint a partner, and as a result, agree to more than they're comfortable with on the fly.

Unfortunately, this can lead to regrets and hurt feelings and might sour one or both people on the idea of parties or threesomes altogether.

So decide in advance what's on the table for any potential visit. Here are some things to consider:

- Watching other people have sex.

- Having sex with each other in a private space.

- Having sex with each other where other people can watch.

- Flirting with other people together.

- Flirting with other people separately.

- Playing with other people together.

- Playing with other people separately.

- The kinds of people you might play with; men, women, nonbinary people, couples, etc.

- Safer sex boundaries and barrier use.

And although check-ins during a party can be tricky, they're not impossible, and they're an important step. Even if something comes up that's within the boundaries you've discussed, make time to check in with each other before moving forward.

For example, if you've agreed that playing with other people is on the table, and someone approaches you and asks about play, make sure you take a moment to step outside or find a quiet area to discuss with your partner before proceeding. Just because playing with other people is an option, it doesn't mean every potential person will be a good fit. And it's important to step out of the situation to have the conversation, so you don't have the pressure of the other person listening while you discuss.

While it might feel risky to step away and come back, anyone worth playing with will support what you need to feel safe and comfortable. If they require a snap decision without giving you time to think or talk, they're likely a bad fit in other ways, too.

Privacy

Some people are so open about their sex lives they publish books about it, others don't want it talked about beyond the people they're actually having sex with. Where do you fall on that spectrum?

If privacy is important to you, this is something to consider as part of your negotiation. Are you all going to tell your friends about the hot time you had, or are you keeping these memories to yourself? If you don't want to be outed as a threesome-haver, be sure everyone involved knows that.

If you're sleeping with people who have other partners, there's a good chance they tell those other partners what they've been up to. Again, if privacy is a concern, ask that the partner be told this should stay private, or see if sharing activities without names is an option.

Play parties and kink spaces often follow the motto that what happens there stays there. But that's in a perfect world. If you're checking out a public space, see what their website has to say about things like a photo policy. Most spaces don't allow phones or photos (but may have an official house photographer), but check to make sure their policies align with your needs.

Of course, at public events it's also possible you'll run into friends or coworkers. My stance is usually that if you see them there—you're both there—so there's a mutually assured destruction if they try to out you. Even so, that's not an encounter everyone wants to have. Be sure to consider your personal risk tolerance for these encounters before heading out.

Keep in mind that if you go from the occasional threesome to actually dating multiple people, privacy becomes more complicated. It can also become an ethical issue if you're asking another person to hide part of who they are, or if you're hiding them from friends and family.

One benefit of being out as a threesome enthusiast, or about being nonmonogamous, is that it's easier to find partners! If folks know what you're into or available for, they might approach you. If you're private about it, you'll have to do all the approaching.

THREESOME SCENARIOS AND TIPS

First Meetings

If the plan is for a threesome, then all three people need to meet up. And while the idea of a three-person date may seem a little foreign, it can ultimately be the same as any first date you'd go on with one person.

Like any first date—especially those arranged on the internet—you want to look out for everyone's safety and comfort by meeting in a public place. Daytime coffee or tea is always a good choice if it works with everyone's schedule. If you're meeting in the evening, people often opt for a bar, so just decide if drinking is within your boundaries for the date, especially if there's possible play the same night.

Hopefully you've already decided if going home together the same day you meet is an option, because that will inform when and where you meet. You may have more flexibility when planning the date if it's not going any further this time around.

Consider options that come with some kind of activity. Whether it's pinball or arcade games or even pool, having something to do can help facilitate conversation and fill any moments of silence. Seeing how someone plays a game is also a great way to learn about them as a person and potential lover. Are they being cooperative or making things about themselves? Are they being pushy? A little competition really brings someone's personality out.

When you're setting up the date, remember that any kind of bait-and-switch is a big red flag. If you've been talking to a couple and then just one of them wants to meet, that's suspicious. Likewise, if you've been talking to a single person and then they plan to bring a friend or partner, sometimes to "just watch," there is a conversation to be had.

If you are planning on play or sex, especially during a first meeting, consider a club or party space for additional safety. As we've discussed, many clubs have bars or other social areas, so you can still have the nonsexual part of the date there. However if you do want to transition to play, there's space for that too, without having to give someone your address or go home with people you don't know very well.

Very important—don't be pushy! Just because you think the date went well doesn't mean it's going to lead to sex that night— or ever. Make sure the other person or people feel comfortable saying no. Being pushy is not only the wrong thing to do, but it's a great way to turn someone from a maybe to a no. After all, if you're pushy on the date (or by message), why should they think their no would be respected during sex?

Getting the Party Started

So you've found your people, you've done your negotiations, and you're all in a room together. Now what? It can feel hard enough to initiate sex with one person, but with two? There can be double the awkwardness.

One of the best ways to break awkward tension is to make

light of it. Just say out loud that you're feeling nervous or awkward and then everyone can admit they're feeling it too, have a laugh, and move on.

Awkward giggling aside, it can feel tricky to actually move things from sitting on the couch to making out, or to heading to the bedroom. Even if you've agreed you're all there for a threesome, you still need to transition from small talk to sexy talk.

To do this, someone needs to take one for the team and initiate. This can be as simple as saying something like, "How about we move this to the bedroom?" or "May I kiss you?" You can also initiate other forms of touching first, like suggesting you take turns giving massages to each other.

You can even share how you're feeling at the same time as initiating touch. How about, "I'm feeling nervous but I'd love to kiss you." Or if you're the third with an existing couple, you could say something like, "It would be really hot to watch you two kiss." Usually once there's some touching or kissing, everyone remembers how to have sex and things start flowing in a way that feels comfortable and natural.

Even with two people, trying to read cues and guess what someone is up for is risky business. With three people it's basically impossible. So prepare to have to suggest things out loud, with your words, and also to ask each time you want to change activities.

If one person in the group has more experience with threesomes, it can even be part of the negotiation in advance that they'll take charge of the situation.

Even if you've done a thorough negotiation in advance, it's a good idea to cover key points right before you get down to business. And starting this conversation is also a great prelude to starting sex.

Try something like, "So, you said you like spanking?" And

voila! You're talking about the sex you're about to have, while also having a chance to reaffirm likes and dislikes.

It's also a good idea to confirm boundaries about barrier use (like condoms and dental dams) and make sure everything that was agreed upon is on hand. Keeping lube, condoms, gloves, and anything else you're going to use within arm's reach will help avoid the awkwardness of going hunting for supplies once things are hot and heavy.

And while most of us keep these items in the bedroom, maybe in the nightstand, try to think about everywhere sex might happen. I've heard of people forgoing condoms in the heat of the moment because things got hot and heavy in the living room. So if your date is starting on the couch, just put a decorative box on the coffee table with some supplies in it. That way you won't need to break the flow to go looking for them.

Three-Way Massage

There's a reason I keep using massage as an example—it's a sensual activity we can share to give and receive pleasure, and the communication required translates well to the communication we need during sex.

To use a three-way massage as an introduction to a threesome, decide who's going first, with the understanding that everyone will take turns. Then decide on an amount of time—maybe ten minutes—and set a timer. Have a negotiation about styles of touch and if any body parts are off limits, and then get started.

The simplest version of this is to cycle through who is getting massaged for ten minutes each. Hopefully by the end of that half hour, you've all gotten comfortable enough with touching each other to transition to the bedroom. But there are some additions you can make as well.

You can try practicing a form of nonverbal communication by how you position your arms. The person receiving the massage keeps their hands by their sides when they want the massage to stay tame, lifts their arms out to their sides if they want it to ramp up a little, and raises their arms above their head if they want all areas of their body touched, potentially with a sexual component, depending on your negotiations.

The arms, and intensity, don't have to move only one way, You can raise and lower your arms as many times as you want during your time period, to keep adjusting the intensity of the massage.

This exercise serves a few purposes. First, the same as any massage, it gets everyone comfortable with touching and being touched. But second, and importantly, it gets everyone comfortable with giving and receiving direction about what forms of touch and play are happening. Doing this exercise will help people learn to give and receive feedback, and also make it feel safer to do so. As you cycle through more and less explicit forms of touch, you'll see that transitioning from one to the other and back again doesn't have to ruin the flow, or ruin anyone's good time. And that's an important thing to remember once you've moved to the bedroom.

Another exercise to try is simply using your words to make requests. As someone is being massaged, they make a request of one or two of the other people, and those people say thank you. As the request is being fulfilled, there's also the option to modify the request. That could go something like this, "Sam, would you please squeeze my shoulders?" And then, once he's doing it, "Could you do that a little harder?"

Getting used to making requests and giving specific direction is going to make the sexual play a lot easier. But most of us don't get a lot of practice doing this. So it can be really helpful to set the tone at the beginning of the evening that asking for what you want is encouraged and celebrated.

Focusing on Inclusion

Don't let someone in your threesome become the third wheel. Unless one person explicitly states they just want to watch, try to keep everyone involved at all times.

There are a lot of ways to include someone in the moment, even if they aren't the star of a particular activity. Sure, given the logistics of sex, sometimes one person might have less of a role, but that doesn't have to be the same as being left out. Simply putting your hand on the third person's body or making eye contact can go a long way. A third person leaning in for kisses while the other two are engaged in penetration can also be incredibly hot.

Another great way to participate is by helping guide the motion of one or both of the other people. Is someone thrusting their hips? Put a hand or hands on them, and help guide the motion. Someone performing oral sex? You can do anything from petting their hair to pulling their hair/pushing their head, depending on what dynamics you've negotiated.

Need more ways to involve yourself in the action? Try asking, "That looks like a lot of fun, can I be next?" Or, "That looks really hot, can I join in?" Or "Can I kiss you while you're doing that?"

Feeling left out can be incredibly vulnerable and can trigger fears of not being wanted or desired. In the face of those feelings, asking to be included can seem scary. Try to remember that everyone was excited about the idea of a threesome and everyone wants you to be there. But if simply diving in feels easier than talking, try stroking someone's arm or back. These kinds of touches can be really nice during a threesome, as they reinforce the "more hands and more sensations" dynamic. Also, a touch like that can sometimes prompt the person to turn and touch or kiss you in return.

You can always take matters into your own hands (literally) and start touching yourself. Either using hands or toys, you can snuggle in beside the other participants and masturbate with a personal live sex show right in front of you.

On the flip side, if you notice that someone is less involved, try to give them something to do. Ask for kisses, or ask if someone wants to switch places so you can all take turns getting attention. Ideally everyone will ultimately get what they're hoping for, so swapping out every so often doesn't mean missing your chance—it just means more forms of play and maybe more anticipation.

It's also okay to take initiative! It's easy for people to get carried away or distracted during a threesome—there's a lot going on! If you go into it expecting to be left out, that expectation can be self-fulfilling.

If there's a moment when you're feeling ignored, see if there's a way you can dive back in. It's far more likely that a particular activity is distracting, and you're not being intentionally left out. Chances are the other two will be delighted to welcome you into the mix.

It's also okay to take a little break and just watch. One of my favorite things about threesomes is getting to watch a partner from angles I don't usually get to see. It can be incredibly intimate and hot to watch your partner with someone else. Even if you're not usually a voyeur, see if you can take pleasure in getting to witness these intimate acts, and pause long enough to really enjoy this experience you're having.

If none of these solutions sound like a good fit, examine whether it's about being left out or maybe just feeling done. It's okay to call it quits, either for yourself or for the whole group (depending on what's been negotiated around this). On the other hand, sometimes a bathroom break or a trip to the kitchen for some water or a snack is all it takes to fortify yourself for another round.

Center of Attention

Being the center of attention is often a love it or hate it position. Some people simply can't get enough attention or stimulation, and other people hate the idea of being in the receiving role. This is helpful information to know about yourself, and your partners, before diving into a threesome.

Why might someone be the center of attention? Maybe the threesome is in honor of a birthday or anniversary or other celebration. Or maybe one person is the tie between the other two—such as in a *V* triad. Or maybe that's simply the way sexual attraction shakes out.

Read on to find lots of options for positions that center one person. But what about the dynamics? If someone is being centered, it's a good idea to make that the explicit understanding. It should probably come up during your negotiation to make sure that's what everyone wants.

The person being centered should also be ready to give feedback and direction. This is even more important than in two-person sex, because now you've got three people trying to coordinate their efforts. This is also a great dynamic for the other two, or the *givers*, to engage in some cooperative camaraderie. Again, don't be afraid to use your words. The more you can assign jobs to people, the easier things will flow.

Check-Ins During Play

Threesomes are not for the "talking ruins the mood" crowd. Even if you're with an established partner and feel like you've got a routine down, this is a whole new ballgame. Not only is there likely to be someone in bed with you that you haven't had sex with before, this may be a new experience for you and a partner, too. So existing patterns and habits won't cut it.

Asking "Is this okay?" is better than nothing, but it doesn't give you a ton of information. Yes, we want to make sure everyone is okay at all times, but that's also a low bar. Not only that, but the question comes with some unintended pressure for the answer to be "yes."

Even if that's not how you mean it, remember that people are generally worried about other people's feelings, and may have tendencies towards people-pleasing. In that context, there's pressure to say yes when asked if you're okay, unless things are really horrible.

Try questions like, "How do you like to be touched?" and "Is there anything that would make this better?" In general, open-ended questions will get you the best information, but they also put people on the spot. People who aren't used to talking a lot during sex will often do better when given a choice between two things. In the context of a massage, that could be a question like, "Would this feel better harder or softer?" In a threesome, or any sexual context, you could ask, "Would you rather I go down on you or use my hands?"

When giving a choice between two options, not only does the other person have to do less thinking, but it can feel easier because there's no wrong answer, and neither choice seems like it will hurt the other person's feelings. What I mean by that is, if you ask if something is okay, you want the answer to be yes. You want your partners to be enjoying themselves, and the person you're asking knows that. But if you're asking about oral sex vs. hand sex, that's a win-win. There are no bad answers, and your question doesn't suggest a preferred response.

It's also a good idea to offer a break every so often. Yes, anyone can ask for one at any time—but sometimes that feels difficult to do. To make it easy on everyone, try to suggest a break every thirty minutes or every hour. Or between any big shift in activities. It doesn't mean play has to stop for the evening, but it's a good idea to take bathroom breaks and get some water, anyway. It can also be a good time to check in and to see what activities people are interested in next.

Be ready to have different responses than you usually do. Kinds of touch that are usually a turn-on might be distracting. Activities that you aren't usually in the mood for might seem like a great idea. This is part of why you need to keep checking in with each other and with yourself. Your body might not be responding in the same ways it usually does, and you might not even notice until you're asked.

Check-ins are also important for giving positive feedback to everyone else. There's a good chance everyone's at least a little nervous—from the usual sexual jitters to wondering how the different dynamics are going to play out. So offer reassurances where you can. If you're enjoying something, say so! If something is hot to watch, speak up.

Especially if there's an existing couple in the room, there's a good chance everyone is going to be waiting to see if jealousy is going to kick in, or if everyone is having a good time. So if you're part of a couple and you're loving every minute of it, find ways to give encouragement. Say things to the new person like, "It's so hot seeing you touch my partner." Or say to your sweetie, "I'm so turned on seeing you kiss someone new." You'll find ways to say it in your own voice, just remember that everyone is eager for positive feedback.

Selfishness and Generosity

Try to reframe the idea of being selfish or greedy. *Greedy* is often thrown at people who have multiple partners, and it's a common insult hurled at bisexual folks. It implies that love or sex can be in short supply, and that some people are taking more than their share. But none of these things are a zero sum game.

The same is true for the word *selfish*. A little selfishness can be a good thing! Our culture shames selfishness so much that people don't realize they're allowed to take care of themselves or stand up for their own interests. But what you really need to be careful of is that you're not looking out for yourself *at the expense of anyone else.*

So be selfish. Just make sure you're encouraging other people to be selfish too.

In fact, with threesomes, it can be helpful if someone leads the charge. So if there's something you want or something you're excited about, say so! Getting your fantasies started can help get the ball rolling, and that's good for everyone. Just make sure that you consciously shift focus to include other people, unless it's been negotiated that the threesome is all about you.

One of the best tips for any kind of sex, including threesomes, is to focus on generosity. At any given moment, is there something you could be doing to bring pleasure to someone else? Something you could say? Or do with your hands or mouth? This ends up working out for everyone, because if each person is being as generous as possible, everyone's pleasure will be centered.

Believe it or not, selfishness and generosity are not mutually exclusive. We can be selfish in ways that don't harm anyone else and we can be generous in ways that don't harm ourselves. In fact, when we're looking out for ourselves, we have more to give to others (just like putting your own mask on first in an airplane emergency drill).

Plan for a Second Threesome

If you've been thinking about having a threesome for a while, you've likely got a long list of things you want to try. And realistically, you're not going to be able to do them all in one encounter. Try to simply enjoy the experience you're having, knowing you can do it again sometime.

This is also a helpful outlook to take if you're feeling a little left out, or like someone else is getting the bulk of the time as the center of attention. Just like with any sex, sometimes one person's pleasure ends up front and center. And that's okay, as long the overall relationship or series of encounters seem balanced.

If the threesome isn't feeling exactly how you'd hoped, ask yourself if you need to fix it right now, or if it's simply giving you ideas for what to propose for next time.

Imbalance of Attraction

Human beings are far too complex to expect three people to all have the exact same level of attraction and chemistry with each other. Does that mean a threesome won't work? Of course not.

While everyone has to get along and have some degree of attraction, that doesn't mean it needs to be a perfect balance. Everyone just needs to be into it, whatever that means to them. And people can have different reasons for being aroused or interested. Maybe one person isn't super into the third for themselves, but really likes seeing their partner with someone they're excited about, and that's reason enough to be in the experience.

What's important is making sure that no one feels left out or undesirable because two of the people are really hitting it off.

Giving Lessons

A threesome can be a great opportunity to give or receive a lesson in a sexual skill. While this needs to be approached delicately to not step into comparison territory, if everyone is feeling comfortable, there is a lot of learning potential.

If you're going to try using a threesome to learn something new, make sure it's framed as an entirely positive thing—a chance to explore and have fun—not as an insult to someone's existing skills. This is about play and exploration, not putting anyone down for their current experience level or skill set.

This format can work well if someone is new to a particular kind of sex, or a particular kind of genitals. I had a sweet threesome with some friends of mine, a man and a woman, where the woman was curious about sex with other women but hadn't had many chances to experiment. After lots of kissing and snuggling, I ended up being the demo model while the man gave her a lesson on hand sex.

He would show her how he was using fingers inside of me, and then she'd try to do the same thing. Not only did the touch itself feel good, but the vulnerability of someone learning a new skill can be a beautiful thing to share. It can also lead to a playful and exploratory atmosphere that allows for lots of talking and laughter, where it's okay to say "whoops" or to try the same thing several times.

It's also helpful to frame this as playful exploration time. Once we call something sex, or even a threesome, that's when assumptions come into play. We have a mental script for how that will go, or what outcomes we're looking for (like orgasms for everyone.) But there are many other ways to interact with multiple people that can be fun, sexy, and satisfying.

Sex Games

You know those games they sell in the bachelor/bachelorette sections of the sex shops? While generally pretty silly, a threesome or group sex scenario can actually be a good time to bring them out. There's nothing quite like having dice to roll or cards to pull to help shake you out of a threesome lull or some momentary awkwardness. It can also help to do something absolutely ridiculous to break any tension that has built up and to remember that this is supposed to be fun and playful.

If you'd like to play some games of your own, here are a few ideas.

Sexy charades—Describe what kind of sex you'd like to have without using any words at all. Just gestures. As a bonus, once someone guesses correctly, you can all act it out together.

Sensation games—Pull items from around the room or around the house and blindfold one person. Then have them guess which object is being used at any given time. Try anything from ice cubes to hairbrushes to create a variety of sensations. Playing a game like this that involves touching can be a great way to break the ice and get things flowing more smoothly.

Strip tease—Pull out your favorite playlist and take turns doing a strip tease or lap dance for each other. You'll feel awkward at first, but it gives you an "excuse" for clothes to start coming of, and people will quickly be into it and stop being self-conscious.

Truth or dare—Play nice! If you're going to try this one, take advantage of the format, but no mean tricks. Make sure you negotiate the parameters of the game before you start. For example, maybe all the truth questions are about favorite sex positions, ways you like to be touched, and sexual highlights from your past. And maybe the dares stick to things above the waist—taking off a shirt, kissing someone on the mouth, neck, or chest . . . things that still count as breaking the ice.

Sexy trivia—Find a set online or make your own questions. Ask about sex scenes from tv and movies or songs with especially risqué song lyrics. You can ask questions about sex scandals from the news and even famous legal cases that have shaped the way we view sex today. People are bound to get answers wrong, and that's a great chance for a bit of laughter and lighthearted teasing. Or maybe you even add a strip element to the game. Each wrong answer loses you a piece of clothing.

Hide and seek—No, I'm not suggesting someone curl up in the antique hope chest. In this version of the game, you hide an agreed upon object. Maybe a small piece of cloth or a feather, etc. Person one gets to hide the object somewhere on person two, while person three isn't looking. And then person three has to find it. Make sure you discuss what areas of the body are on and off the table for this. And then, within your negotiated limits, enjoy a sexy frisking.

Toys, Props, and Supplies

With multiple people comes multiple levels of stamina. So it's a safe bet that some people will start to wear out before others.

Toys can come in handy if one or more people are winding down, and someone else is still looking for stimulation. They're also a great way for people to stimulate themselves, or for a third to lend a hand while the other two are involved.

Adding toys to the mix can also open up options for far more sexual positions and fantasy scenarios. For example, a strap-on is a fantastic addition to a threesome. There are such a wide variety of strap-on options that you can even get strap-on harnesses that fit over thighs, over boots, or across the chest. They add a great deal of flexibility to the ways bodies can combine. Strap-ons that accommodate a penis can be helpful when the person with the penis wants to give penetration but doesn't have an erection.

If you're buying your first harness, you may want to go to a shop where you can try one on. You can also find companies online who will design a harness to your exact measurements. There are many different styles, and you'll want to find one that's the most comfortable for you.

For example, you can get harnesses in both a thong and jock-strap style. Personally, I prefer the jockstrap style, with an open back. Not only are the straps flattering to the ass, but they allow genital contact if you want to receive touch or penetration while you're wearing the harness.

Consider your material of choice. While many harnesses come in leather, that also makes them more expensive and more difficult to clean. Leather is porous so it can never be truly sanitized (and trying will harm the leather.) If you're going to be playing with multiple partners, you may want to get a nylon, fabric, or vinyl harness so it can be more thoroughly cleaned.

Another useful threesome toy? Dildos! Even if no one is wearing a strap-on harness, dildos are great to have around. Make sure your dildos are made from silicone or another nonporous, sanitizable material. Toys made from glass or stainless steel are easy to clean, making them a good fit for use with multiple partners.

Dildos are available in a wide range of styles, from ones intended to look realistic to ones made in wild colors and even glitter. It can be nice to have a couple different options on hand. Consider smaller toys if anal penetration is going to be one of the activities.

Here are some other toys to consider.

Butt plugs—When you're getting a toy for anal play, make sure it's well made and intended for that purpose. You want something that is made in body-safe material and also has a flared base or wide handle. Make sure the base is wider than the widest part of the toy, and also that the neck of the toy (between the wide part and the base) is long enough for your body to close around it.

Butt plugs come in a variety of shapes and sizes and can be a great addition to play with one, two, or three people. Because of their shape and wide base, they can be put in place and then left hands-free, so you can focus on other things. All the while, they provide some extra stimulation.

Prostate toys—While butt plugs provide general sensation, toys made specifically for prostate play are shaped to provide directed stimulation. These toys will usually have a curve to their shape, to better reach the prostate. Some are dildo or vibrator style, and will need a hand on them to keep them in place, and some, like Aneros toys, can be used hands free. The hands-free options are especially nice for group play because, like the butt plug, you can put the toy in place and then focus on other activities, all while experiencing the extra stimulation.

Vibrators—Vibrators are a great toy to have on hand no matter who the players are. A cordless, wand style toy is my personal go-to. While the wands might seem large and intimidating at first, their long handles make it easier to reach the right spot from a variety of positions, no matter who is wielding the toy.

Vibrators are an especially nice toy for a third to wield, in order to help out with sex that might otherwise be duo focused. Anything from missionary to doggy style positions can benefit from some extra stimulation. A vibrator is also a great option for engaging in safer play. With gloved hands and toys like vibrators and/or dildos, you can have all the sex you want without any skin to skin or fluid contact.

Vibrator add-ons—Wand-style vibrators come with a number of additions to help them do more specific jobs. They come with silicone covers for different textures, dildo-style attachments, and also sleeve-style attachments for use on penises.
Wedges—Wedges, like those made by Liberator, can help make many more sex positions possible, or just more comfortable.

They're sturdier than a pillow, so they can raise your hips (for oral sex, for example) without squishing back down. They also make wedges that have slots to hold a vibrator, so you can lean over one while receiving penetration from behind, or any other number of positions.

Waterproof blankets—Whether you've got a squirter in the mix or just want easier clean up, it can be helpful to throw down a waterproof blanket before play. That way no one is stuck in the wet spot, and you don't need to change your sheets before going to sleep. They come in a variety of sizes and colors, so you're bound to find one that works with your decor.

Lube—A sex must have! From solo sex all the way to an orgy, good lube is an essential supply. But not all lubes are created equal. Read the ingredients to make sure everything is body safe. Unfortunately, many commercially available lubes, like those you'll find at the drug store, contain ingredients that aren't good for you. For example, you'll often see glycerin as one of the ingredients, and that's a sugar derivative—meaning it's likely to give people with vulvas a yeast infection. If you've got a sex-positive sex toy store in your area, check them out and talk to their employees. Or check out one of the trusted online shops from the resource section.

Another thing to look out for is compatibility with toys. Silicone lubes can't be used with silicone toys, as they'll degrade the material. So stick with water-based lubes when using silicone toys.

Kink toys—Everything from rope to floggers to paddles to whips to feather ticklers! If this is your cup of tea, grab a book specifically about kink or check out one of the online retailers from the resource section to see what grabs your eye.

The great thing about adding kink to a threesome is it gives you even more possible combinations of bodies.

Masturbation sleeves—A masturbation sleeve is something that's made to slide a penis into. They come in a wide variety, everything from a TENGA EGG, which is a thin sleeve you hold with your hand to provide a different sensation and texture than you can achieve with your hand alone, to things like a Fleshlight, which come in their own case.

A wide variety of styles are available. Some allow varying degrees of pressure to be applied, and some have a hard case. They have all different shapes of openings as well as internal textures.

Some of the handheld sleeves can even be a nice addition to a hand-assisted blow job.

Cock rings—Cock rings come in a number of styles, but the basic idea is that they go around either the base of the penis, or both the penis and testicles, in order to trap blood in the erection. Many people also simply enjoy the sensation of the tight squeeze. Cock rings are also available with a bullet vibrator to provide either stimulation to the clitoris of someone being penetrated, or additional stimulation to the wearer.

Making Sure Everyone Is Satisfied

How do you know if everyone is satisfied? You ask! Don't assume someone has had an orgasm, or as much touch as they'd like, without verbal confirmation. All too often one person climaxes and then just assumes the party is over, and they transition to snuggles—or worse, hop out of bed to shower or get dressed.

It's important to not only hear what someone's needs and desires are before getting into bed, but to make sure those needs and desires have been met before hopping out. Sure, not every fantasy is attainable, and sometimes things don't go as planned. But within reason, you should make sure that everyone is feeling good before the activities come to a close.

A threesome (or any group sex) is a marathon, not a sprint. Keeping that in mind, pace yourself. If you know that after an orgasm you're done for the night, try and hold off until everyone has gotten what they want from the experience before you climax. And if you are worn out and need a break, see if you can be a supportive audience member if the other two are still going strong.

Simultaneous orgasms are rare enough for two people, and are simply not going to happen for three. So be prepared to shift focus as everyone gets what they need to leave the experience happy.

Maybe this means someone masturbates while the other two people touch and kiss them. Maybe this means someone has toys used on them. It's understandable if things are lower energy by the end of the night, but there are mellow ways to share pleasure.

I can't emphasize this enough: make sure no one is made to feel "needy" for having needs. This is true in all sex, and doubly true with threesomes, group sex, or when trying new things. Basically, any time someone is feeling extra vulnerable, it's important to honor that vulnerability with gentleness.

Need more suggestions for how to keep going when your energy is waning? What about getting comfy and participating with dirty talk, or tossing suggestions at the two people still playing? You could even grab a book of erotica to read aloud, or find some hot porn to play for the whole group.

Threesomes and group sex can definitely be more exhausting than twosomes, but making sure everyone feels taken care of and leaves happy is the best way to ensure that there are more threesomes in your future.

The End of the Night

Of course you've already pre-negotiated how the night is going to end. You've decided if there's going to be an overnight, and if not, who is staying where. So maybe your end of the night is everyone curling up in the same bed (with someone in the dreaded middle spot), or maybe somebody, or everybody, is going home.

Just like at the end of any date, you'll want to exchange some pleasantries. And just like any date, it's a bad idea to lie in an attempt to be polite. Don't say "let's do this again sometime," if that's not really what you want. You can always just say thank you.

Assuming everything went mostly well, try to end the evening on a positive note. Thank everyone for being there and for sharing themselves, and if there's something that stands out from the evening, now is a great time to mention it. You can share what your favorite moment was or something that was especially hot for you. You can thank someone for helping you have a new experience.

These end-of-night kindnesses are a good idea whether you're laying the ground for a second date or simply sending people home feeling happy about the experience.

Engaging in New Kinds of Sex

As we've discussed, having a threesome could mean your first chance to explore a brand new kind of sex. That could mean sex acts you've never tried before, or it could mean sex with new kinds of people, or it could even be both at the same time! Here are some tips to help that go smoothly.

First, make sure everyone in the room knows what your level of experience is and what you're hoping to try. Also, share how you're feeling. If you're nervous, say so. If you want to go slow, say so.

Next, make sure the person you're trying the new thing with is ready to give you a lot of direction and feedback. Some amount of feedback is always necessary with sex, even if you're not trying a new thing. Every body is unique, and you'll always need to learn the way a new person likes to be touched. But especially if the acts or the kind of person are new, you'll need not only direction for its own sake, but for reassurance. Ask questions like, "Do you like this?" and "Does this feel good?" Along with open ended questions like, "How do you like to be touched?" It can also be helpful to ask for guidance with a question like, "Will you show me what you enjoy?"

If you're having sex with a person of a gender you've never had sex with before, remember—we're more alike than different. Start by thinking about how you like to be touched, and how your other partners have liked to be touched, and from there just ask questions.

When it comes to operating genitals you're not familiar with, don't panic. I promise, they're not as different as you think. In fact, we're all made from the same stuff—just arranged a little differently. Whatever you're touching, start gently and then ask for guidance. Questions like, "harder or softer?" or "faster or slower?" apply no matter what part of the body you're working with.

I know from my clients that performing oral sex on unfamiliar genitals can be particularly intimidating. People also seem to use this as a "test" for whether they're really into a particular gender. First of all, you never have to prove your sexuality. But I understand the impulse. I still remember the first time I went down on another woman. I really wanted to see how into that—or not—I would be, as though that would say something about my identity.

But because of that eagerness, I was doing it with the first person I had a chance to do it with rather than someone I was romantically interested in. It turns out that genitals on their own aren't necessarily exciting for everyone. So don't put too much stock in your reactions to a particular activity. Not only that, but plenty of people simply don't care for performing (or receiving) oral sex, regardless of sexuality or situation.

All that said, here are some oral sex tips:

▶ Enthusiasm counts more than technique. People like to see signs that you want to be there, and that you're enjoying what you're doing.

▶ Make eye contact.

▶ Make noises that indicate enjoyment.

▶ Tell the person that they taste/smell/look good. We're all self-conscious about these things.

▶ When going down on a penis or strap-on, remember that deep throating skills are a nice party trick, but not at all necessary for pleasure.

▶ Using your hands isn't cheating! If you're going down on a penis, hold it in your hand for stability and extra stimulation. If you're going down on a vulva, you can take breaks to swap out with your fingers, or combine penetration with your fingers (after asking first!) with oral stimulation of the clit and labia.

▶ You don't need to keep going until the other person has an orgasm. It's totally fine to switch up activities at any time, or to ask them to help out by touching themselves.

▶ If you don't want cum in your mouth, that's okay! Just ask for a heads up, and you or they can finish by hand.

Remember that one of the beautiful aspects of a threesome is the ability to try new things. And it's okay to not enjoy every new activity you try. Think about it like going to an ice cream shop. You get the taster spoon of a bunch of flavors before you decide what goes in your sundae.

POSITIONS

The Nitty-Gritty

What does it look like to add a third person to sex? We've talked about a lot of logistics to get you there, but what do you actually *do* with a third person in bed?

When thinking about positions, remember that there are a wide variety of ways to be the giver or the receiver. Think beyond penetration, and when penetration is involved, think beyond a penis.

For example, imagine the missionary position, perhaps the most well-known sexual pose. There's no reason that has to be a cis woman on her back and a cis man on top—it can be people of any gender on either side of the equation. Maybe the person on the top is wearing a strap-on. Or maybe the person on top is simply reaching a hand between their bodies and penetrating or stroking with fingers. Rethink everything. Penetration can be vaginal or anal, and external stimulation can be for any genitals at all.

Here are some ideas for how to arrange three bodies, with the above flexibility in mind.

Sweet Kisses

Remember at the beginning of this book when we talked about expanding our definitions of a threesome? One of the best and easiest ways to have a threesome is by keeping things simple.

Imagine any two-person sex position you're used to, then imagine it with the third person kissing one or both people. Yes, it can really be that simple. Maybe that means missionary sex with the third person laying alongside the bottom and kissing them, while occasionally leaning up to kiss the top. Maybe it's three people laying alongside each other, touching and kissing. Maybe it's just a three-way make-out session that lasts for hours and hours.

While your threesome fantasies may include some varsity-level positions—and may even require some specialized athletic training—when it comes down to it, just having a third person in the room is going to feel exciting.

Mutual Masturbation—For Three

Mutual masturbation is always a great way to share intimacy and excitement—while also getting exactly the kind of touch you want, and having the safest sex possible, with yourself.

Mutual masturbation is frequently suggested as an option for two people, but why not for three? Find positions where everyone can see everyone else. Maybe spread around the bed, leaning up against the headboard and footboard. Make sure everyone has enough room to move, and keep some lube and toys within reach, too.

Now, everyone gets to touch themselves in whatever ways they enjoy most, while in full view of everyone else. You get the turn-on of seeing other bodies and other people's pleasure, while also maintaining a little bit of space. This can be the main event for the encounter, or it can be a great way to start or finish a threesome.

At the start, it can work as incredibly sexy warm-up. Everyone gets to see what they're soon going to get to touch, while also getting themselves turned on for the activities. Not only that, but you can watch and learn what kind of touch each person enjoys.

At the end of the evening, it can be a lovely way to wrap up and make sure everyone is getting off. Or getting off again. This way everyone leaves happy, without the pressure on anyone to perform or figure out exactly what works for anyone else.

If you give this a try, I bet you'll find yourself coming back to the hot memories of people touching themselves in front of you time and time again.

Side by Side

Maybe you start side by side on the couch—the classic date-night position—but with an extra body. This works especially well if the person in the middle likes a lot of attention and/or if the other two people don't want too much close contact.

The people on the sides can touch and kiss the person in the middle, and the person in the middle can use their hands on both parties. There are a couple of ways to do this, either all sitting side by side, or with the middle person turned around to face the other two. Each version will give you different amounts of access and will offer different logistics. If you want to go all the way to hand sex in this position, you'll need to consider your angles.

While all sitting side by side, the person in the middle can have a hand between each other person's legs, providing a variety of stimulation. If fluid transfer isn't a concern (or if swapping out gloves) the person in the middle can also switch focus from one side to the other, while both people on the ends keep kissing and touching the middle party.

For external stimulation—for example, giving hand jobs to people with penises—all three facing forward can work very well. That's a great angle for the person in the middle to work from. If the person in the middle wants to provide penetration—whether vaginal or anal—turning around and facing the people on the couch will make that a lot easier.

Another option is for the middle person to easily move between the other people's laps, straddling them and kissing while the other person has a fantastic view and also free hands for touching. The exchange of lap dances can easily last a whole evening.

This playing on the couch dynamic can be especially nice for a first threesome, because sticking to the couch can feel less serious, and therefore less intimidating, than moving to bed. Even if you do all the same things on the couch you'd do in a bed, the environment can feel more casual.

Doggy Plus Oral

A threesome classic, this is the doggy style you're used to, but with a third person in front of the bent over person. Most often, the bent over person is receiving penetration while also performing oral sex. This position is ideal for someone who likes to be the center of attention or who likes a lot of stimulation.

This is also a great option for all three people to be receiving genital stimulation at once. If there's worry about someone feeling left out, this position keeps everyone intimately involved—and involved in a way that can potentially lead to an orgasm.

While any combination of genders and bodies can try this position, in pictures or pornography you'll often see this with a man penetrating a woman in doggy style, with another woman lying on the bed. The woman in the middle being penetrated from behind is able to go down on the woman in front of her.

If the woman in the middle is bisexual or pansexual, this can be a best-of-both-worlds scenario. It can also be a good position if the person in the middle is exploring sexuality, and wants to try going down on a new kind of person for the first time.

While performing oral sex under distracted conditions might seem less than ideal, the distraction can actually be a benefit. For one thing, if you're getting fucked, you're going to be less in your head about the details of what you're doing with your mouth, which can help with performance anxiety. And being jostled around also means you can't aim for precision. That helps make it more about the overall experience than the details.

If the person doing the penetration has a lot of stamina, or is wearing a strap on, it can be nice for the other two to swap positions in order to take turns with the various forms of giving and receiving.

Doggy Sandwich

Imagine two people in roughly the missionary position, with a third person behind. The person in the back is penetrating the person in the middle, while the middle and bottom person make out. The bottom two people can also be using hands and toys to stimulate each other, but I'm actually a fan of sticking to kissing in this pose.

While it might sound boring at first read, because not everyone's genitals are involved at once, it's actually a very intimate position for the two people on the bottom—being face to face, having eye contact, and kissing makes this a good choice for people who are sweet on each other.

When I was in a triad, this was a favorite position of mine. I liked being the one all the way on the bottom, on my back. With my girlfriend on top of me, I could look into her eyes and kiss her. I could feel her body pressing against mine, and feel the movements of her being pressed into from behind. I could also easily look over her shoulder to my boyfriend behind her, and with a bit of a stretch he and I could kiss as well.

This position is a great opportunity to enjoy the communal aspects of a threesome. To enjoy the closeness of three bodies pressing together, even if not everyone is engaged in an overt sex act that might get them off.

Spit Roast

A porn mainstay, the spit roast is similar to the doggy plus oral position above, but in this variation the person in the middle is being penetrated at both ends, either with penises or strap-ons. This means being penetrated from behind (that's the doggy style) and giving a blow job in front. Like for all of these positions, the penetration can be vaginal or anal.

This position is particularly intense for the person in the middle because each person thrusting drives the other side deeper. It's a good idea to be comfortable with deep penetration and deep throating if you're going to get vigorous in this position—if not, make sure the people on each end know to go easy.

This position allows for an easy change-up if the people in the front and the back want to switch places. Depending on preferences, someone can even swap in for the middle role, too.

While the classic version of this position has the person in the middle on their hands and knees, you could certainly change things up by having the middle person on their back. The people on each end will just have to adjust their angles a bit. In fact, if you can do this at the edge of a bed so the person on their back can tip their head back off the edge of the bed, that makes it even better for deep throating—having your head tilted back at that angle makes it a straight shot down your throat.

Remember that whenever your mouth is full—especially if you aren't in control of the position—it can make check-ins difficult or impossible. Try to keep at least one hand free, and maybe on the hip of the person penetrating your mouth, so you can "tap out" as necessary, or at least get their attention for a check-in.

Eiffel Tower

Honorary mention for being arguably the most entertaining threesome position, an *Eiffel Tower* is a spit-roast with the addition of the two upright partners high-fiving each other over the middle partner's back, or even doing a double high five, therefore making the point of the Eiffel Tower.

As absurd as this sounds, it has become *a thing.* Surely with the help of internet porn and sex-based listicles, this is a position many sex savvy folks will be familiar with.

One of my favorite artists[7] did a series of Kama Sutra Bunnies—I have a print of the whole lineup in my living room. But I have the original drawing of the bunny Eiffel Tower in my bedroom, and it makes me smile every day.

And although this is perhaps more of a joke than an actual sexual position, it's something I've engaged in multiple times. I've been the center of the tower, with two people high-fiving over me, and I've been one of the high-fivers, too, while wearing a strap-on.

Sex is often silly, and even more often it's playful. And this is a good thing! It's wonderful to bring moments into the room that can add levity and give everyone a chance to smile or even laugh. Remembering that sex is playful can take a lot of the pressure off, and doing something outright silly is a great way to intentionally release that pressure valve.

Double Penetration

Another threesome porn classic, the most common form of double penetration is two penises (or dildos) in the same hole. But this can also refer to simultaneous vaginal and anal penetration.

The simplest way is to add a third person to your standard

---

7   Follow @nywnart—Bronwyn Schuster—on Instagram to experience the bunnies yourself.

straddle arrangement. The third gets behind the top partner—like adding doggy style—and the person in the middle is penetrated by both people.

Keep in mind that if you're trying this with two penises, it's likely trickier than you realize to coordinate two erections, especially when you couple pressure to perform with the position itself taking some finagling. Be ready with a plan B, whether that's one or two toys or simply switching to another position.

Another thing to know is that if you've got two penises in the same hole, and they're both wearing condoms (which they probably should be!), you're at much higher risk of a condom breaking. Condom on condom friction is trouble, so if you're trying this, make sure there's a lot of lube in the mix, and that you're ready to take on that additional risk.

In a variation on double penetration, I once had some birthday sex that involved two penises in my mouth at once. One of the people was a serious partner, and we didn't usually use protection for oral. The other fella was a friend and more casual partner. To avoid the two of them having direct skin to skin contact of their penises—for the sake of STI safety— my casual partner wore a condom and my serious partner did not.

You could try a similar solution in your own double penetration scenario, if you're fluid bonded with one of the players. If you're unfamiliar with that term, being *fluid bonded* means you exchange fluids with that person. This means engaging in penetrative or oral sex without condoms or other barriers.

Even with these considerations, remember that a logistically challenging position is going to be harder on a condom, and also may make you less likely to notice if something has slipped—because there's a lot going on and you'll be distracted.

★ ★ ★

The intensity of double penetration means the receptive person needs to be very aroused for it to feel good. It can be helpful for the receptive person to lend a hand, literally, by touching themselves or using a vibrator externally to make sure they stay turned on enough for this to be fun. Helpfully, arousal diminishes the pain response.

Double Straddle

In this position, one person is laying down and two people are on top—one mounting a penis or strap-on, and the other sitting on the bottom person's face. The face sitter can be facing either direction, but it's especially nice to face the other top partner so you can make out.

The two people on top have a lot of freedom of movement, and also have their hands free, so it's easy to spend time exploring each other's bodies or wielding sex toys to provide some extra stimulation.

For the person on the bottom, it can be a great way for them to have their senses overwhelmed and to feel completely immersed in the experience. They also have hands free and can reach up to hold the hips of the person sitting on their face. (This allows them to tap out as needed!)

I had a great time in this position when I was at a sexy house party. A married couple I was friends with were having sex in a straddle/cowgirl position, and I was invited over to play with them. They suggested I sit on the man's face while his wife was straddling his hips, being penetrated.

At this point the fella on the bottom didn't have a lot of freedom of movement, but that didn't really matter. While I was on my knees, I was able to stay upright enough to not entirely smother him—although he sure wasn't worried about that. He had his hands up to hold my hips and kept pulling me further down onto his face. And while he couldn't give me verbal check-ins from that position, his hands on my hips always let me know how he was doing, and that he could still breathe.

Meanwhile, his wife was riding him and taking charge of most of the movement on her end. He was able to thrust his hips forward to some degree, but most of the riding action was her responsibility.

Perhaps best of all, she and I both had our hands and mouths free, so we were able to have an incredibly hot make out, and play with each other's breasts, while also receiving pleasure from below.

Tag Team

Here's another option for one person who wants to give and receive at the same time. Someone lays on their back—perhaps at the edge of the bed. Another person is standing and penetrates person one (vaginally or anally, with a penis or strap-on), while the third person sits on person one's face—facing forward or back.

It's similar to the double straddle, but with one person standing, so the standing person has more leverage. Standing is also a lot easier on the knees, which can make this position last longer.

Especially if there's a strap-on in the mix, this can be a nice option. If the person wearing a strap-on doesn't also have a penis, they're likely not as used to being in the thrusting position—and that takes a lot of muscles! You may find yourself hurting in some new places the next day, after your first strap-on adventure. So standing up can be a much easier way to go.

If the bed isn't quite high enough, or you're aiming for anal penetration, it can be nice to add a wedge under the receptive person's hips, too. This will make for a much more favorable angle for penetration.

Double Oral

Just like the name sounds, double oral is two people performing oral sex on the third. You've probably seen this in porn, with two women performing a blow job, but any configuration of genders and genitals works.

Giving a shared blow job can actually be really hot (including giving a strap-on blowjob!) It's a great view for the person receiving, and the two people giving can take breaks to kiss. This is also a fantastic position for people who like sloppy oral sex. Sharing oral sex on a vulva also works, but needs a little more turn-taking to make room.

If you like this idea but want a little more personal space, you can also have someone standing or laying on their side while the other two perform oral sex from front and back—either a blow job or cunnilingus in front, and rimming in back.

If part of your threesome involves someone exploring with a gender or genitals they are less familiar with, the double oral position is a great option. This way, the person with experience can guide the newer person, showing techniques and also providing support.

At a recent play party, I had a hot experience engaging in this position. Once we'd finished with snacks and small talk, we settled in around the living room for an opening circle. That's a chance for people in the room to get to know anyone who's new to them. It's also a chance for people to share their name, pronouns, safer-sex info, and their likes and dislikes, as well as a great time to figure out who you might want to approach or play with.

During the opening circle of this party, one of the attendees—we'll call them Kris—said they'd love to receive a strap-on blowjob. I immediately took note. Not only was Kris a super cute nonbinary babe who'd caught my eye, but I love giving strap-on blowjobs. As the circle continued, another person, an occasional play partner of mine, Mia, mentioned they enjoyed giving strap-on blowjobs . . . and a scene began to form in my mind.

As soon as the circle broke up, I asked Mia if she'd be game for helping me give a strap-on blowjob, and she was an enthusiastic yes. We approached Kris together, and they were thrilled with the idea and slid their leather harness on.

There's a special kind of dildo[8] that allows for suction from a blow job to be transferred to the person wearing the toy, and luckily, Kris had one of these on hand. Once strapped on and ready to go, Kris stood while Mia and I knelt at their feet.

I know some people don't understand the point of a strap-on blowjob because there isn't the same kind of direct feedback you get with a bio penis, but let me assure you, there's plenty of worthwhile hotness.

For starters, Kris had two babes on their knees, eyes cast upwards. With both hands free, Kris was able to pull our hair or slide fingers into our mouths. And with our free hands, we were able to hold Kris's hips and reach up to stroke their arms and chest. Being face to face, Mia and I were able to take breaks to kiss each other, or to kiss with the silicone cock between our mouths.

If you enjoy a messy blowjob, then a shared blow job might well be for you. Switching back and forth between givers, and sometimes even sharing, leaves a lot of opportunity for drool.

And if you're using a strap-on, because of the mechanics of the toy, you actually suck far more than you would with a bio cock, and that means you get the hot visual of hollowed out cheeks plus the sounds of slurping and suction.

Although it was only the three of us playing, and we were lost in our own world for quite a while, we were in the middle of a play party. A few folks were sitting nearby and watching the

---

8   Aptly called the B.J. Dildo by Form Function LLC.

action. So not only did we have our own hot scene, but we had the additional turn-on of an audience.

It's also worth noting that, aside from the risks of swapping spit—no riskier than any kissing—this whole hot encounter was essentially free of STI risk. There was no genital to genital contact and no mouth to genital contact. Only contact between mouths and between mouths and the silicone toy.

Yet, to my mind, this totally "counts" as both sex and a threesome. While no one had an orgasm, everyone was turned on and having a wonderful time. We carried on for quite a while, and in addition to the sucking and licking, had a lot of opportunities to play with the dynamic between the three of us.

Kris was topping both of us and engaging in lots of hot dirty talk, playfully calling us names and asking if we liked having their cock in our mouths.

Playing with a strap-on is a great reminder of how much of sex isn't about the alignment of bodies, but is about the dynamics and the energy of the play. Looking up at Kris, with their silicone cock in my mouth and their hand in my hair, was just as intimate as any sex act you might do skin to skin.

This was also a example of three friends coming together to play, with no existing couples in the mix. While Mia and I had played together before, it was always in the context of parties and other shared experiences. And we both only knew Kris socially.

The Oral Switch

The counterpoint to the double oral position, the oral switch works particularly well with one person kneeling and two people standing. The person who is kneeling can switch back and forth, giving oral sex to the other two. This works for any genital configuration, but is a bit easier if the standing people either have penises or are wearing strap-ons.

Keep in mind that if you're going back and forth between two bodies to perform oral sex, those two people are becoming fluid bonded by way of your mouth. So if swapping fluids isn't on the table, this should be done with barriers in place.

This same position can work for hand sex, or for mixing hand sex with oral. Rather than having someone wait their turn while the other is being pleasured, the kneeling person can keep a hand up, stroking and touching. This way, everyone is involved at all times.

While it might sound submissive for the person on their knees, they also have a great deal of control of the situation. So you have a lot of choices about what dynamics you might enjoy in this scenario. The two standing people can "use" the kneeling partner, perhaps adding hair pulling and dirty talk. Or the two standing people can be at the kneeling partner's mercy, waiting for their attention. Of course, the position can just as easily be power neutral if that's your preference.

This position is very flexible in terms of how, or if, the standing people interact with each other. If they're hoping to keep a little distance, this position makes that easy. But if they're also into each other, it's very easy for them to be kissing and touching as well.

Oral Sex Train

Is oral sex your favorite? You can arrange three bodies so that everyone is giving or receiving oral sex. The easiest way is to mirror the double straddle, but with all oral rather than penetration.

In one of my many silly sex adventures, I ended up in this position while drinking a cup of tea. There were four of us playing, but two of us were on a break. I was sitting off to the side, watching one fella go down on the other. The man on his back invited me over to sit on his face, and I pointed out that I was taking a tea break. He told me to bring the tea with me, so I did! Is that kind of ridiculous? You bet. But it was also lots of fun. Not only did I get to enjoy my tea, but someone was going down on me, and I had a great view of a hot blow job happening in front of me.

Daisy Train

The daisy train is somewhere between the oral sex train above and a classic 69 position. It's also a bit tricky logistically. For this position, you arrange yourselves into a triangle so that everyone is going down on someone while someone goes down on them.

Much like the 69, I think this position is better in theory than in practice, but it can be a good option if you're determined to have everyone equally involved at all times. Just remember that when your neck gets tired or your hips start to cramp, it's totally fine to take a break and then switch to a more comfortable pose.

Chain Link

This position builds off of doggy style, but you simply add a third person in the back. Generally, the third person is also providing penetration, either with a penis, a strap-on, or a handheld toy.

This position requires a fair amount of coordination, because if people are thrusting out of sync, the whole system can fall apart. But if you find a nice rhythm, this can be a lot of fun, especially for the person in the middle who can penetrate and be penetrated at the same time.

The Math Equation

Imagine a 69 and then add one. The additional person can penetrate either person, but the easiest option is to position the 69 as top and bottom, and for the third to assume a doggy style type position behind the top of the 69. Just be careful when it comes to balance. The person doing the thrusting can easily knock someone off their game. So be sure to have solid footing for this position. In fact, it can be best if the penetrating person is actually standing. Then their hands on the other person's hips can add some helpful stability.

If the 69 is side by side, the third can add on in a spooning position.

The Reverse Straddle +

Someone lays on their back and someone straddles them—but instead of facing that person, they're facing their feet. Typically they'll be riding a penis or strap-on. Benefits of this position include the chance to get different angles of penetration and the ease of movement it allows to the person on top. And if the person on the bottom particularly enjoys a backside view, this can be a special treat.

So where does the "plus" come in? Here's where we get to some of the varsity-level threesome logistics. The extra person camps out between the bottom person's legs, and therefore between the top person's legs too.

If the person on top leans back, this bonus person can have access to go down on both people at once. If the bottom person has a penis, the bonus person can lick their testicles.

This position can be made a bit easier to access for the third person if the person on the bottom has a wedge or some pillows to raise their hips up off the bed. Then the bonus person won't risk such a serious neck cramp.

If you like the idea of this pose but don't want as much of a workout, the third person can also chip in with hands or toys while they have their easy access spot between the other two people's legs. Bonus: if they're using hands, they'll be free to kiss the upright person at the same time.

Spoons

Speaking of spoons, while it takes a bit of lining up, you can also make like three spoons in a drawer, with the person in front being penetrated by the person in the middle, and the person in the middle being penetrated by the person in the back.

Whether you have two or three people, the spoon position is a good one for sweet and tender sex, and it's also easy on the body if you need a comfortable position. This one has a lot of opportunity for cuddling and wandering hands.

The person in the front can even flip around to face the person in the middle—if you're willing to get your legs all mixed up a bit, this can work for penetration as well, and now you can add a little kissing, too.

Bukkake

Bukkake generally describes multiple parties ejaculating onto one person. But you can be flexible with what you're considering ejaculation—squirting counts too! This often feels hot for people because of the taboo aspect—or, if it's part of how you're playing, an element of consensual humiliation.

In a threesome scenario, ejaculating onto someone's body (like on their breasts or chest) can be a nice option because, as long as you're willing to hop in the shower after, it's easy to clean up. And from an STI standpoint, it's safer than coming inside someone's body or mouth.

Whether you're going for simultaneous ejaculations or simply coming on a person's body one at a time, it can be a nice option because it generally involves masturbation. That makes it a great way for someone to take their pleasure into their own hands—literally—while the other person or people are participating by creating a sexy view, as well as a target.

★ ★ ★

A partner and I had a threesome with a friend of mine, and we learned that she particularly enjoys directing where someone ejaculates. She appreciates the control it gives her, while on the practical side it also gives her a heads up.

As we played, my partner asked her both if and where he could come, and she instructed him to come in her hand. I never would have thought watching someone present an open palm could be so hot.

The Voyeur

We've already established that voyeurism is one of the pleasures of a threesome—so why not make it explicit? Position a cozy chair in full view of the bed and let one person just watch.

Maybe the watcher is touching themselves, maybe not. Maybe they're giving instructions, or maybe they're simply watching the show.

This position also has a lot of kink potential. The person in the chair can be blindfolded so they can only hear what's going on, but not see it. This can be ramped up a bit with a little additional teasing, with the other two coming over to touch or kiss the person in the chair every so often. Or even putting something against their mouth for them to kiss or lick.

The person in the chair could also be gagged, so they can watch but can't comment on anything they're seeing. More hot teasing potential here.

If you know what you're doing, you can even add bondage, tying someone to the chair so they're "forced" to watch everything happening in front of them. Again, with added teasing if you desire.

You can also throw sex toys into the mix here, especially those with a remote control. What if the watcher has a vibrator inside or against their body that's being controlled by the people in the bed? Maybe they need to beg for permission to orgasm.

If you're kinking up your three-way, consider the power play potential of who's doing, and who's watching, at any given time.

This is also a good option for people who have decided to take the plunge into three-way play, but still want to move slowly. Whether it's the couple or the single person who's new to threesomes, either having an audience or taking a front-row seat is a great way to experience the hotness of a threesome, while still keeping some training wheels on.

The Handmaiden

In this position, someone lays back against the headboard, propped up like they're going to watch TV in bed. Then someone else lays back against them—using them like one of those sit-up-in-bed cushions. And then the third person mounts the second person, in a somewhat modified missionary situation.

The person all the way in the back may be able to get some hot friction action by pressing up against the person laying against them, but that isn't the main thrill of the pose. Instead, the emotional and power dynamics are key here. The person in the middle can be playing proxy for the person in the back (as in the book where this position gets its name) or the person in the back can be holding the middle person down.

You can further play with power by deciding if one person is being ignored. Maybe the person on top doesn't look at the middle person, but instead makes eye contact with the person in the back. Or maybe it's the person in the back being ignored. See what combinations of power play do it for you.

The person in the back also has free hands for other forms of fondling, or toy holding, if they'd like to chip in. And depending on your exact lineup, there are a variety of opportunities for kissing.

Taking Turns

While people seem inspired to find positions where everyone is getting off all at once, sometimes it can be easier—and even more fun—to simply take turns being the center of attention.

This is the usual pattern with my regular couple fling. It's not that there's never more than one thing going on at a time. But we work our way through participants pretty methodically when it comes to making sure everyone, well, comes.

In a recent tryst, the wife got to be the star of the show first. She was on her back on my bed as I went down on her. Her husband moved between kissing her and touching her breasts and fingering me and touching my ass.

His touching felt perfectly supportive—adding to the arousal for each of us—without pulling focus away or demanding attention. Sometimes she'd reach up for his cock to play with it by hand or to lead it to her mouth.

After going down on her, I switched to using fingers and toys. When she was ready to have an orgasm, she helped by touching her clit while I was inside her. Everyone knows their own body best.

Next, she pushed me down and pressed one of her thighs between my legs. We grinded together while alternately leaning in to kiss each other and reaching up to touch her husband, who was by our side, on his knees.

After I had an orgasm, it was his turn to be the center of attention, and she and I shared his cock between our mouths, sometimes pausing to kiss each other, and sometimes gazing upwards to make eye contact with him. Eventually, she was on her back again, and he was masturbating onto her chest.

While not everyone was in focus at all times, by the end of the evening everyone had had their turn in the spotlight, and everyone had gotten what they wanted from the encounter.

CHAPTER

17

BDSM AND THREESOMES

How Does Kink Affect a Threesome?

Folks who are savvy at threesomes and folks who are savvy at kink have (at least) one thing in common—they're better than average at communication. But when you combine kink dynamics with multiple people, there are some things you want to be aware of.

Remember that both adding people and adding kink elements can up the stakes, and up the emotional intensity of an encounter, so you want to be ready for that. As much as you'd communicate for either of these scenarios alone, double or triple your communication efforts when putting them on the table together.

Talk about *everything*. Make sure you're unpacking any assumptions you have about how things will go, and make sure everyone is on the same page. Refer back to chapter 14, on negotiation for a refresher if you need to.

How will power dynamics work? How will power dynamics affect how you communicate and check in during your play? What toys are you going to use? Are you mixing both sex and kink?

This is a great time to pull out some yes/no/maybe lists[9] that cover both sex and kink to make sure you've thought through everything you do and don't want to do. A yes/no/maybe list is basically a menu of sexual and kinky options, so you can think through what activities you might be up for. You can then compare lists with the people you want to play with. You'll find a threesome-specific list in the resources section of this book to get you started.

If this is both your first threesome and your first exploration of kink, go slow and take it easy. Try something simple like spanking or light bondage, or maybe some light power play with giving and receiving orders. Kink can get very intense very fast, so give yourself a gentle first time around and then come back for more if you're into it.

Roles and Power Structures

If you're joining people who engage in kink, are there any explicit BDSM dynamics already at play? Are the people involved in a negotiated dominant/submissive relationship? If so, how does being around those dynamics feel to you? And where will you fit in? It could be a good idea to read up on kink a bit—everything from how-to books to erotica—to see if this holds an appeal for you.

If you're going to be participating in someone else's BDSM play, it's also a good idea to have a clear picture of what those dynamics entail, so you can be sure whether it's your cup of tea.

Do the people have honorifics they use as part of their play? Some people use terms like *Daddy* or *Master*. So find out in advance if that's the case, and check in with yourself about how that makes you feel.

If the idea of exploring dominance or submission appeals to

---

9   You can find a simple version in my first book, *Tongue Tied*, or a downloadable version on my website at www.stellaharris.net/kink.

you, a threesome can be a fantastic chance to get both a live example and hands-on guidance. Maybe in the course of the threesome you learn to give a spanking, or how to use a flogger. Or maybe you get to experience being tied up (with people you trust!).

Kink can feel easier to explore when someone in the room has a lot of experience. So whether you're joining a kinky couple, or adding a kink-experienced third to the mix, there are countless possibilities.

Kink Parties

We've covered kink parties a bit already, but here's an area where they'll really shine. It can be easier to dive into a bit of kink at a party than to dive into public sex. And some parties even offer *tastings*.

A tasting in a kink context is a chance to try out a toy or sensation with someone that the venue or party host trusts. So, just like a wine tasting, you can try a few things to see if you like them. The idea of a tasting is that it is limited in both time and intensity. So maybe a quick spanking, or a chance to get flogged on a cross.

Whether you go to a party solo or with a partner, you may find people who like sharing their skills. And asking to see what a particular paddle feels like can be easier than asking for sex!

If you're at a party solo and you see a hot couple you'd like to play with, watch what they're doing together. Be sure not to interrupt a scene while they're playing or engaging in aftercare. But once they're done playing, or when they're socializing, introduce yourself. If you liked what you saw, say so. And maybe ask if they'd be willing to show you a thing or two.

If you're there as a couple, it works the same way. Maybe you see someone giving a spanking and you're dying to try it. Wait until they're free and express your interest. If you're there with someone, maybe one of you wants to experience the spanking and the other one wants to learn how to do it. A lot of people at kink events are more than happy to share a few tips or techniques. Or maybe you simply want to watch your sweetie getting spanked by someone else, or you want to help out by holding your partner down or kissing them while it happens. Because kink parties offer a wide variety of ways to interact, there are a lot of experiences you may be able to share.

Shaking Up Couples' Dynamics

When people find themselves partnered to someone on the same side of the power dynamic—such as two dominants or two submissives—sometimes sex gets tricky.

On more than one occasion, couples have found their way to my office because they each identify as submissive, and deciding who will take the lead during sex has become a point of stress. Or, less dramatically, certain fantasies just aren't being fulfilled. Adding a third person to the mix can be a great way to shake up kink or BDSM dynamics.

A few years ago, I got to play with this exact scenario. I was dating another woman, and while we were both switches, we ended up rather submissive around each other, and we'd get trapped in, "I don't know, what do you want to do," territory for frustratingly long periods of time. While I'm usually a fairly take-charge kind of person, something about my dynamic with her just short-circuited my usual tendency to take initiative.

Finally, at a kinky play party, we found a solution to our problem. We found someone else to take the lead for both of us! We talked to a trusted friend about what we were looking for, and he was only too happy to oblige.

So she and I ended up lying face down, side by side on a big bed, and our friend went through his whole toy bag on us. We were whipped and paddled and flogged and caned—all the while we were giggling and holding hands, making eye contact, and having the experience together.

We found a way to share an intense experience, while both being in the bottom or submissive role. And because we had kink at our disposal, we were able to do the whole thing without negotiating sexual contact with a new person, or worrying about STI risk. (Though of course kink play comes with its own set of risks, and we did negotiate our kink play.)

Whatever your dynamics, adding another person can shake things up. Whether that person tops both of you, or you two top them, simply interacting with another person brings out different parts of your personality. There are myriad options to explore.

Possible Combinations

When splitting up the power exchange dynamics in a threesome, you can have two people topping or two people bottoming. (And you can always switch things up as you go!)

If two people are topping, they can share responsibility for restraining the third and providing intense sensation, like impact play (spanking, etc.). Maybe they use rope or cuffs, or maybe they simply pin someone's arms down. It can be especially hot to simply hold someone's arms over their head while you look down into their face. Maybe at the same time the other person is spanking them or flogging them.

Or perhaps you like the idea of more gentle play, like exploring sensation. You can use items from around the house like ice cubes, pieces of fur or silk, feathers, or anything with a scratchy texture (even long fingernails). If the bottom is blindfolded, every sensation will be more intense, because they won't know what the object is, or what's coming next.

If two people are bottoming, the person topping has a lot of options. They can tie two people together and watch them struggle and wiggle while being tickled or poked. Or they can direct their own personal sex show, telling the other two what to do and how to do it.

Playing with power and control is a classic form of kink, and it doesn't require any special tools or toys. And while it does require some confidence and know-how, there's less of a learning curve than for many other forms of BDSM.

You can have one person in charge the whole time, or you can choose to change things up at any time. Let the person in charge direct or choreograph the other two, or have the other two ask permission before they're allowed to do anything.

Try experimenting with edging (getting close to orgasm and then backing off) or orgasm control, either with people touching themselves, or by playing puppet master and controlling when and how they touch each other.

Not only is playing with power hot, but the increased talking and direction also works as a check-in. Nothing happens by surprise, and people always have the option of saying no, or negotiating for an alternative.

Good Guy/Bad Guy

A fun dynamic that can play out if you've got two tops and a bottom, or two dominants and a submissive, is that classic combination of the good guy and the bad guy. Maybe one of the tops is really on your side and is trying to take it easy on you, while the other person's being mean. A set-up like this is ripe for all kinds of playful role-play or dirty talk.

Sometimes this dynamic will emerge from how people naturally relate to each other, and sometimes you'll have to plan for it. You can even draw straws to decide who will end up in each role.

Kinky Threesome

One of the times I got to explore kink dynamics within a three-some was when visiting a long-distance partner. The way we'd scheduled the visit, one night was going to be for just the two of us, and the next night her other sweetie was going to join us. He and I are friends, but don't have a sexual relationship.

In part by focusing on kink elements, with our shared partner bottoming to both of us, the three of us got to enjoy lots of hot play while maintaining boundaries that everyone was comfortable with.

For our planned threesome night, we opted to attend a play party. Going to a party for our play time had a few benefits. Of course there were the socializing aspects, and we got to enjoy the shared sexual energy of lots of people playing at once, many in view of each other. But it also had another benefit—by playing in a shared space, it took the intimacy down several notches.

While playing in public (at parties) can be incredibly intense, it does have a different energy from being alone in someone's bedroom. You get to catch people's eye across the room and smile at the things going on around you. Although the sex can still be intimate, being in a shared space can also help keep things playful.

The three of us claimed a bed and played with ordering our shared partner around. Being submissive, and the center of attention, was a perfect fit for her. We took turns delivering some impact play while the other person kissed her or pulled her hair—or both at the same time. Eventually she went down on her other sweetie while I used a strap-on from behind.

We each got to have our own intimate moments with our shared partner while also enjoying a playful camaraderie with each other. And having kink elements to fall back on helped make that possible.

PERFORMANCE ISSUES

Don't Count on an Erection!

You may have some very specific ideas about what you'd like your threesome to include. But try not to get too attached to any particular outcome. Pressure to perform is one of the best ways to guarantee that an erection either won't show up or won't stay around as long as you'd like. And having multiple people you're trying to please can be some high-level pressure.

For example, if you're aiming for double penetration with two penises, not only is there pressure for an erection, there's pressure for two people to coordinate their erections! That's much easier said than done.

Whatever you're planning for your threesome, have several backup plans and be willing to be flexible. To help with this, make sure your sexual toolkit extends way beyond things you can do with an erection. How do you feel about your oral skills, your ability with fingers and hands, and your proficiency with toys?

One of the best ways to manage erection worries is to simply take the erection (whether it's there or not) out of the game plan.

At least for a long while. Not only is this a great way to manage anxiety and have a sexy good time, but it opens up more positions and more forms of play. And that flexibility will serve you well in a threesome. After all, an erection can't multi-task . . . but maybe you've got two hands for touching two bodies at once.

If you're not used to having sex that isn't penis or erection focused, get some practice with that before your threesome. That might mean whole sexual encounters that never involve your penis, or simply saving penis play for much later in the game than usual.

What happens if you simply focus on your partners' pleasure for a while? Maybe try to give them multiple orgasms, or orgasms from multiple methods of stimulation. If this is out of character, talk to your partner about what you're doing. If someone is very used to a certain pattern in sex, it can be jarring to change the pattern up without warning.

Kevin Patterson also emphasizes this advice: "Taking the pressure of PIV off the table from the start works better. There's no performance anxiety, and you have permission to go with the flow. Getting your hand skills together is really important. Hands don't get soft. I've gotten a better response from people who invite me to group sex situations when I deprioritize my own dick."

Did you know that an erection isn't necessary for pleasure, or even orgasm? While it can feel pretty vulnerable at first to have a soft penis played with, there's a lot of pleasure to be had there, so give it a try some time. You can engage in all the same forms of touch you'd use on an erect penis—for example, performing oral sex. In fact, an added benefit of going down on a soft penis is that it's easier to get the whole thing in your mouth, even if you're not a deep throat fan. You can use a bit of suction to pull the penis into your mouth, and then provide additional sensation with your tongue. Using suction in this way can help produce the same "up and down" motion you might be used to with an erect penis.

Also, remember that erections and arousal aren't the same thing. You can be hard when you're not interested in sex, and you can be super turned-on and not be hard. So there's no reason to let an erection (or lack thereof) dictate what will or won't happen.

If this idea is new to your partner(s), it's worth explaining. Make sure they know that erections are sometimes elusive, and it has nothing to do with how turned on you are, or how attractive you find them. Be sure to reinforce this with lots of compliments as well as praise for other forms of pleasure—like the way someone is touching other parts of your body.

Don't Expect an Orgasm

Sure, orgasms feel wonderful. Maybe you even included having an orgasm in your definition of sex. But orgasms are never a sure thing, and getting too goal focused is a good way to scare them away.

No matter what kind of genitals you're working with, feeling like you're under pressure to have a particular reaction tends to have the opposite effect. With threesomes, the journey is often more fun than the destination. And while it might feel frustrating to not have an orgasm, especially if you're really turned on, getting too focused on that goal can also take your attention off of other pleasurable activities.

Your threesome experience might become fantasy material for days, weeks, months, or even years to come. Who knows how many orgasms you'll end up having thanks to these memories. So don't miss out on the moment if your body isn't doing exactly what you're hoping for.

If you're feeling frustrated or stuck, see if you can shift the focus to another part of your body, or better yet, focus on someone else's pleasure for a while. You might be able to circle back and have an orgasm later, but even if you don't, you'll be having a better time in the moment than if you stick with something that isn't working for you.

Also, don't be afraid to chip in and touch yourself. We know our own bodies better than anyone else can. So if you can touch yourself, or use a favorite toy, while other activities are going on, that might be enough to get you to the orgasm you're looking for, if that feels like an important part of the experience.

Skill Set Anxiety

No one has perfect confidence when it comes to sex—or when it comes to anything, for that matter. So it can be especially nerve-racking to think about your sexual skills being compared to someone else's in real time.

But guess what? That's not how it tends to work. Everyone does things differently, but different doesn't necessarily make any style better or worse. We can enjoy a change of pace, or some variety, without actually preferring someone else's technique. Do you have a favorite flavor of ice cream? Do you ever like to mix it up and try something else? Or better yet, have a two or three scoop sundae—the threesome of the ice cream world? Of course you do. And that's not a judgment on the ice cream. That's because we like variety and novelty.

If anything, we tend to learn our partners' bodies over time, so we're often pretty good at doing what they enjoy. A new person may have the benefit of novelty and excitement, but they won't know about *that thing* that drives your partner totally wild.

Try to remember that new and exciting isn't the same as better, and simply ride the wave of increased arousal from the novelty. And if a new person is doing something that seems to work especially well, ask them to show you how they're doing it! A threesome is the perfect time to learn some new skills.

It's a shame that more of sex isn't taught through hands-on learning or demonstrations, so take advantage of the opportunity to learn in real time.

Comparisons and Insecurities

Everybody is different. And every body is different. We tend to frame things as better or worse, but differences can simply be variety. And variety is one of the great reasons to engage in threesomes.

When you bring someone else to bed, you're going to see someone whose body is different from yours and/or your partner's. People will have different sized breasts and different sized penises, and will be different heights and weights. People will also have different levels of experience, different skill sets, and different amounts of stamina.

It's far too easy to get into the trap of comparing yourself, and other people, to some theoretical cultural ideal—and that's a great way to have a miserable time.

Before bringing extra people into the mix, it's important to do some honest reflection and figure out what your personal insecurities are. Everyone has them, and that's okay. But if you're not aware of them in advance—and not prepared to deal with them when they crop up—then you're more likely to take those insecurities out on other people.

If you're part of an existing couple playing with a third, it's important to be transparent about your insecurities so that your partner doesn't accidentally trip on emotional landmines.

For example, if you've always wished your breasts were larger and you end up bringing in a third with a voluptuous DD cup, you may find yourself comparing bodies when you should be enjoying a sensual smorgasbord. And if your partner is unaware of your insecurity, they may compliment the new person on their breasts in a way that hurts your feelings, or even highlights differences.

Here's the thing—all breasts are amazing and fun to play with. Having breasts of different sizes and even textures in the room is one of the magical experiences to be had in threesomes. Enjoying and celebrating a variety of bodies can be a beautiful thing.

I speak from experience when it comes to comparisons—I've been guilty of this myself. A few years ago, I had a partner who loved threesomes, and we had quite a few of them together. He was also (like me) into rope bondage. A number of the people we played with were more flexible than me. I have a fused disc in my spine, and that really limits how I can bend—in a way no stretching routine can fix. So when we'd play with someone he could basically fold in half, I'd feel like that made the other person more fun to play with. He could do more of the fancy rope bondage positions we'd learned in classes with these other people than he could with me.

Here's how I talked myself out of that spiral. I asked myself if rope was the only thing we enjoyed together, and of course it wasn't. I asked myself if we'd still have a solid relationship even if we never did rope together again. And of course we would have. And that helped me let it go. Even if these other people were "better" at being tied up, that didn't threaten my relationship.

And of course there's more to it than that. Being more flexible doesn't mean "better." What about their reactions to his touch, or their ability to communicate their experience? Those are vital parts of a rope bondage scene, too, and those are areas where I am confident.

This same partner was also very into (giving) anal sex. And that was something we did together sometimes, but it's more of a special occasion thing for me. My body isn't always up for it, and it takes a lot of warm up for me to get there. So when we were having a threesome with someone who was seemingly just ready to go, I'd feel like that highlighted a failing on my part.

But again, I could ask myself the same series of questions. And of course our relationship didn't hinge on anal sex any more than it did on rope bondage.

Not only that, but because we were engaging in threesomes, I could still be a part of him getting his anal sex desire met. And thanks to some assistance from my strap-on, I was able to be intimately involved—by being half of the double-penetration team.

Eventually, I not only stopped comparing myself to the other partners, but I began to be grateful to them. Grateful that, because of their participation, my partner was able to engage in all the things he was interested in—even when they were things I couldn't or wouldn't do very often. Not only that, but knowing he was able to satisfy those desires elsewhere, I no longer felt like I needed to push myself to do activities that weren't my favorite.

Another place where comparison can spoil the fun is comparing the reactions your partner is having with a new person to the reactions they have with you. Maybe it seems like they're moaning louder, or having an orgasm faster—but none of that means the sex is better.

Threesomes can be hot and exciting—that's why you're doing it, right? And when the whole experience is a heightened state, it's easy for reactions to seem a bit more dramatic than usual.

Not only that, but your sweetie might also be playing things up on purpose, as a way to validate and encourage the new person. We're often louder when we want our partners to feel like they're doing a good job—our sex noises are a great way to provide feedback! So remember there are a lot of reasons someone might sound a little different from what you're used to.

Your mantra for your threesome experience: different doesn't mean better.

THREESOME INTERLUDE

The Surprise Threesome

I was attending an out-of-town conference and sharing a room with a friend and occasional lover. We were theoretically both people who are awesome at communication—sometimes that can backfire. Sometimes when you're good at something, it actually gets easier to skip the basics.

And somehow this friend and I had managed to entirely skip any negotiation around the logistics of room sharing. Was this trip like a date for us? Was sharing a simple matter of convenience? What if one (or both) of us wanted to bring someone back to the room?

We also failed to negotiate anything about how our arrivals or departures would work. And I realized that mistake immediately upon arriving at the hotel.

I checked in at the front desk, got my key, and went up to my room. I simply unlocked the door and let myself in—and found my roommate in the middle of sex with another mutual friend and occasional lover.

I have kind of a routine when it comes to work travel. I like a lot of alone time. I use my hotel room to recharge and to hide from people between activities. Immediately upon entering the room, I realized that an introvert rooming with an extrovert could get complicated.

My friends greeted me enthusiastically and invited me to join them on the bed—and in sex. Given that a quiet entry clearly wasn't going to happen, I hopped in bed with them. If you can't beat 'em, join 'em?

We played with a few configurations, but largely ended up in the *doggy plus oral* position. The other woman and I took turns going down on each other while the fella was behind, and penetrating, the person performing oral sex.

Luckily, we were all friends and lovers, but no combination of us was a couple—so that limited the emotional complexity or fall out from the situation. Ultimately we all had a satisfying and sexy time—but even so, it's bad form to surprise someone with sex of any kind, and especially a threesome.

SAFER SEX

Having the Talk

Any time you're negotiating sex with a new partner, it's a good idea to have a check-in about safety. If you're part of a couple opening up for the first time, you might be a little rusty at this.

If you're part of a couple, keep in mind that while it might feel scary to add someone new to the mix, no one wants to be treated like Typhoid Mary, so talk about risk and safety as it pertains to *everyone*, not just what the third might be exposing the existing couple to.

Regardless of configuration, everyone who is sexually active should be getting tested for STIs on a regular basis. Ideally you have a doctor or health-care provider who is well versed in sexual health and safety who you can be open with about your activities. If that's not the case, look into Planned Parenthood or other local clinics.

If you're going to ask someone else about their testing history, it's important to have yours to share as well. So even if you've been monogamous or single for a while, if you're getting back in the game, consider getting tested.

There's no such thing as getting tested for "everything." Each doctor and clinic, at least in the US, has their own idea of what a full panel of testing is. Usually this includes gonorrhea, syphilis, chlamydia, and HIV. Most doctors have stopped testing for HSV (herpes) on a regular basis because the most used tests aren't very reliable, and it also isn't considered a big health risk.

Infections can be location specific, and that means if you're having oral or anal sex you need to be swabbed in those areas, as an infection wouldn't appear in a urine sample. Oral and anal swabs are not standard procedure at most clinics, so you'll need to ask for them. Be ready to firmly and confidently advocate for yourself.

When talking testing and safety with potential partners, be sure to share what you were tested for and when, as well as asking for the same information from your potential partner. Some people don't just want to talk about testing, they want to see the actual test results. This can take the form of a printout of results, or even results sent online or via apps designed to do this job.

While you're checking in about safety, it's also important to talk about birth control—if that's relevant to any of the participants involved. Remember, even if you're using condoms, they aren't a sure thing, so it's nice to have a backup method of birth control on board.

While it can seem like these conversations may be awkward, or just not sexy, they are a great way to make sure everyone is looking out for each other. And having this conversation is a good way to find out if the people involved will be able to have other tricky conversations that might come up.

Before you have the talk, figure out what answers you're hoping to hear, so that you're not making a judgment call in the moment. When faced with a cute person you'd like to have sex with, the temptation is too strong to bend your own boundaries and feel bad about it later. So make an agreement with yourself—and your partner(s) if you have them—about what kind of safety protocols work for you.

For example, do you want people to have been tested in the last three months? Six months? The last year? What do you want them to have been tested for?

You may also want to know how many partners someone has had since their tests and what their barrier use practices are. Also, whether they have these conversations with everyone they have sex with. If someone is taken aback by this conversation, there's a good chance they never do it. I find you learn as much about someone by *how* they have this conversation as you do from what they actually say.

Once you've decided to move forward, you also need to decide what safety precautions you want to take for your encounter. What activities will you engage in and what barriers do you want to use? Whatever you decide, it's helpful if multiple people bring supplies, just in case. You don't want your activities to be cut short due to a lack of condoms, or gloves, or other supplies.

Build Your Conversation

Information you might want to cover:

- When you were last tested, what you were tested for, and your results.

- Your relationship status and relationship agreements.

- How you identify your gender and sexuality, your pronouns, and your body part words.

- Sexual encounters you have had since you were last tested.

- Your barrier use practices with other partners.

- Whether you always have safer sex conversations.

Multiple Players, Multiple Boundaries?

Safer sex is always an important consideration, but it can become especially confusing when there are multiple people playing at once. Multiple people can mean multiple layers of boundaries. For example, maybe two people in the bed are fluid bonded, but neither wants to exchange fluids with the third person.

Aside from having different layers of boundaries in mind, when it comes to multiple bodies in a bed, it can get difficult to even remember whose hands or mouths have been where.

Think about it: maybe you go down on your sweetie like you're used to doing, and then you want to kiss the third person—well, now there are fluids on your mouth you may be exchanging. Or maybe you've touched someone else's genitals and then you're going to touch your own, or your partner's. It can be hard to keep track of where your hands have been.

Rather than keep track of different levels of boundaries and where everyone has been, it can be easier to have everyone playing adhere to the strictest level of boundaries at play in the space. Meaning, if there's a couple who usually swaps fluids but doesn't want to exchange fluids with the third, maybe this encounter involves no fluid exchange at all. Perhaps oral sex is off the table, or is done with condoms and/or dental dams for everyone involved.

People in the kinky or queer communities are familiar with the use of gloves for safer-sex, but often other folks haven't heard the idea. While it might sound strange or impersonal at first, gloves are a fantastic way to introduce some additional safety to your sexual adventures.

One approach is for all genital touch to be done with gloves so you can easily switch to a fresh pair for the next person or activity. You can even color-code your gloves so you know which one touches which person. Maybe purple gloves for partner A and blue gloves for partner B. You can also use the color-coding technique to track kinds of play to avoid cross contamination, such as anal play and vaginal play. Or you can even use color-coding to tell different sizes of gloves apart at a glance.

Another way to avoid cross contamination in groups is to dedicate particular sex toys to each person so you don't need to remember what's been used where. Otherwise you might want to use barriers over all of your toys—even for use on yourself—and be sure to swap them between each use.

Barriers and Supplies

Mouthwash—There is some evidence that using antiseptic mouthwash after performing oral sex can decrease the likelihood of oral STI transmission. However, the protection this may give is not nearly certain enough to count on this as your only precaution.

Dental dams—Dental dams don't get nearly enough love, but they make oral sex so much safer! A dam is simply a rectangle of latex that you spread over the area you want to put your mouth on. You can use a dental dam for oral/vulva contact or oral/anal contact. There are even companies making wearable dental dams—meaning dams that you can pull on like underwear and that stay in place hands free. So there's no more excuse about them being awkward to keep in place.

Condoms—The safer-sex classic, condoms are for penises and for any phallic shaped toy. Condoms come in a variety of materials, most commonly latex—but with an ever-growing list of nonlatex options for people who have sensitivities or allergies.

It's also worth noting that condoms come in a range of sizes and styles. You can look up condom size charts online, as there's no standardized sizing across brands. It really is worth finding a condom that fits comfortably. You can also get sample packages from many sex shops or online retailers so you can keep trying options until you find one that you like.

If you're not used to wearing condoms—maybe you've been with the same partner for a long time and you're fluid bonded—you may want to get used to them again before you try them with a new partner. There's enough pressure during your first time with a new person—try not to add even more variables.

Go to a sex shop, or order online, and get a nice sample of condom brands, sizes, and styles. Then start trying them with your existing partner or when you masturbate. Get comfortable putting them on, and get comfortable playing while wearing them. That way they'll be second nature again before you need them during your threesome.

Internal condoms—Sold under the brand name FC2, internal condoms can be worn in a vaginal canal or a rectum. These are a great option for people who have concerns about erections coming and going during play, as there's no risk of the condom slipping off, like there can be with external condoms.

The great threesome hack with internal condoms is that, if you have more than one hole at play, you can have each person wearing an internal condom and the penis can go back and forth! You can't do that with an external condom, as that would still transmit fluids between the two receivers.

Internal condoms can also provide some additional safety from skin-to-skin STI transmission, like HSV, because the opening of the condom covers some of the vulva.

To use an internal condom, you'll need to make sure you're using lube. The condoms also come with an internal ring that's supposed to make them easier to insert. However, some people find them uncomfortable and you can remove them before use. If you're going to use an internal condom for anal sex, you'll definitely want to remove the internal ring first.

Gloves—Latex or nitrile gloves are an incredibly useful tool to have in your safer sex kit. They help make sure that your fingernails won't scratch whatever sensitive tissues they're touching (especially important for vaginal or anal penetration), and they also prevent bacteria from the hands or nails being transferred to a partner. Not only that, but gloves make cleanup much easier. Rather than running to the bathroom to wash your hands several times during sex, you can simply remove gloves and put on a new pair. This is especially important when moving between anal and vaginal play—as cross contamination can cause infections—or when moving between touching two people's genitals.

Because some people have a latex allergy, I find it's easier to just keep nitrile gloves on hand so I don't have to worry about which gloves to use. Personally, I find the black gloves pretty sexy, but I keep different colors for easy, at-a-glance size differentiation. (As a bonus, I always have gloves if I want to dye my hair or do a messy household task!)

Lube—We already talked about lube as a supply to have on hand, but did you know that lube contributes to safer sex, too?

Using lube can help prevent microtears of sensitive tissues, and that in turn keeps you safer, as those tears can allow bacteria or viruses into the body. Lube can also help make sure that barriers aren't experiencing too much friction, making them less likely to tear.

When you're choosing lube, make sure you do your research. Head to a sex-positive store in your area or hit up one of the online retailers in the resource section. You want to make sure you're getting a high-quality lube that has only body-safe ingredients.

Many water-based lubes have additives like glycerin that can cause yeast infections, or other additives that can cause burning or irritation. I like to stick with a simple body-safe water-based lube for all my play. Be especially suspicious of anything that warms up, cools down, or comes in flavors—those are going to have extra ingredients that probably aren't very good for you.

Silicone lube is simpler because it's just silicone. So that's body-safe. The trick there is that silicone lube isn't compatible with silicone sex toys. So you've got to pay attention to what's going where.

You can also get oil-based lubes, but beware—oil degrades condoms and other barriers so they can't be used together. (That goes for things like coconut oil too, which can also have other complications. Stick to things sold and tested as sexual lubricants.)

Safety Tips

If you're going to be having any skin-to-skin contact or swapping any fluids, keep in mind you want your body to be as protected as possible.

While we all want good breath before making out with a cutie, try not to brush your teeth for at least a few hours before performing oral sex. Brushing your teeth can create microtears in your gums, and then you're basically bringing an open wound to the party that you may rub against someone's genitals or genital fluids—placing you at greater risk. So, especially if you're going to perform oral sex (on a penis, vulva, or anus), stick to mouthwash or a mint for before-play freshness.

The same theory holds true when it comes to shaving! If you shave your pubic hair (or get it waxed), try to leave twenty-four hours between your grooming routine and your sex adventure.

Otherwise you could have openings in your skin that make it easier to pick up an infection.

Remember to use a new barrier every time you switch activities. If you're going to be penetrating two people, you need to switch condoms every time you switch partners. If you're switching between anal sex and vaginal sex with the same person, you need to switch condoms. Same is true for gloves and dental dams. They only do their job if they're only used once! Make sure you start with plenty of barriers on hand so you can keep switching them out while you play. And do yourself a favor and keep a trash can next to the bed for ease of disposal.

COMMON PITFALLS

Unexpected Feelings

The first step to addressing any difficult feeling is to name it. Think about your feelings until you have some words for what you're experiencing—is it jealousy, insecurity, overwhelm? Speak up about how you're feeling to your partner(s). Simply pushing down the feeling and letting it fester only makes things worse.

Too often we decide that having an emotion like jealousy or insecurity makes us a bad partner, or even a bad person, and that fear makes us stay quiet. Then we're dealing with shame on top of everything else. The number one way to combat shame is to share what you're feeling. Allow others to hear and validate your feelings and to reassure you.

It's helpful to remember that feelings aren't facts. Maybe you're afraid that your partner thinks a third is more attractive than you. While your fears are valid, and worth recognizing, that doesn't mean they're the truth. Make sure that you can acknowledge your feelings while also recognizing when they're coming from a place of fear, and don't take the voices in your head at their word.

When you're talking to someone about your fears and insecurities, make sure to own your own feelings. These feelings aren't something your partners are doing to you. Don't say, "You're making me jealous." Try saying, "When I see you kiss someone else, I feel jealous." Remember to use "I" statements—that will be more likely to create empathy on the part of the listener. Otherwise you're just accusing them of something, and they're likely to get defensive.

If possible, have a solution or request in mind at the same time. "When I see you kiss someone else, I feel jealous. Would you please kiss me now?" Sometimes it's as easy as getting the attention you're craving.

This can also go the other way—unexpected romantic feelings when things were agreed to be, or expected to stay, casual.

It turns out, feelings are unpredictable. And all the agreements in the world can't prevent them from cropping up. Be ready to have the conversation if someone catches feelings during or after a threesome.

Are you open to having that conversation? Is continuing to see someone an option? If so, would that be separately or together?

Remember that just like equal attraction isn't a given, neither are equal feelings. It's possible that two of the three people will form a distinct connection. While you can certainly decide that's something that won't be pursued, having the feelings come up can still be disruptive.

Safer-Sex Slipups

No amount of negotiation or preparation can safeguard against the occasional accident. Whether it's being forgetful or having a barrier slip or break, things happen.

If you've already had a solid safer-sex talk, you should have a good idea about how the people you're playing with treat safety concerns. In fact, one of the reasons to have that talk is to get a sense of how people will handle accidents if they happen.

If you'd like, you can even negotiate in advance about how you'd like to manage potential accidents. For example, if a condom or other barrier slips off or out of place—what next? Do you put on a new barrier and keep going, or is that the end of activities for the evening?

Either way, it's best to acknowledge what happened, when it happens, and see what everyone needs in the moment. While some people feel comfortable carrying on and addressing things more thoroughly later, sometimes it will break the flow to the extent that the encounter needs to stop entirely. It's also possible that someone will be upset enough in the moment that they need to stop and have a conversation about next steps, or simply be comforted.

Remember that while stopping can be disappointing, if you're careful about people's needs and feelings, they'll be a lot more likely to want to play again another time.

While regular STI testing is always a good idea, some people may want to go in for an additional test if there has been unplanned fluid exchange or skin-to-skin contact. Do your research about incubation periods, and talk to your doctor about your concerns, because you generally won't get an accurate test result within a few days of potential exposure.

If you know the person you were playing with had an STI, and know you were exposed, tell your doctor and they'll likely provide treatment even without waiting for a positive test result.

Jealousy Threesome

Many years ago I explored an intense D/s dynamic with a new partner. It was my first relationship with explicit power play, and it brought up feelings I'd never dealt with before. Being experienced with open relationships, I knew that I didn't default to jealousy. But something about this new dynamic made me compare myself to everyone else this particular partner was playing with.

Making things worse, he was a photographer, too. And while I loved the images he took of me and of our play, he also photographed his other partners. So I didn't just hear about what he was up to with other people, I got to see it too.

One night I made the mistake of checking social media when I couldn't sleep, and I saw that he'd posted pictures of a scene with someone I felt jealous about. She was younger than I was, and somehow I'd decided she was more fun, or a better fit for him.

The pictures showed that they'd been engaging in the same kinds of play he and I had just done the day before. The same toys were being used, and the photo was even captioned with a phrase he'd said to me. I didn't get back to sleep all night.[10]

Soon after that, he organized a photoshoot with me, her, and one other partner/model. We were out in the woods together, freezing our asses off, and making art. After the shoot he invited us all over for tea to warm up. Only the woman I'd been comparing myself to and I were able to stay.

At first, my heart sank. What would it be like to spend time with both of them at once? One-on-one she and I were friendly, but I didn't know what to expect from the combined dynamic. We sat there sipping our tea, and before long he proposed kink play with both of us. I was hesitant at first, but couldn't stand the idea of opting out and having them play without me.[11]

We began a threesome featuring parallel play. She and I interacted, of course, but the kink and sex play was between each of us and him. A *V*-shaped threesome, with him at the crux.

---

10 To be fair, that wasn't a great move on his part.
11 Do as I say, not as I've done!

Adding to the fun, she and I were both blindfolded, so we could hear what was going on, but couldn't see anything.

She and I were on our hands and knees on the floor, and our wrists and ankles were tied together, my left to her right. This kept us so close to each other that we easily felt every movement and reaction from the other person. For example, he would spank her, and I would feel her body moving with each impact and hear the sounds she made in response. I got both the thrill of the auditory voyeurism as well as the anticipation of knowing everything I was hearing would happen to me next.

Even though he was doing the same exact things to both of us, saying the same exact words, I could see how different it was. What he was doing was the same, but the way she and I reacted was totally different. I was well behaved, she was bratty. I followed direction, she acted out. The dynamic couldn't have been more different. By the time the threesome moved from kinky to sexy, I was fully relaxed and turned on.

As we transitioned from one kind of play to the next, he untied us. He knew I was enjoying listening to the play, so he moved her onto the bed first and left me sitting on a bench to the side of the bed, still blindfolded and with instructions to hold still. I no longer had the physical input for what was happening, but I could hear everything. And I was familiar enough with the sound of the Magic Wand vibrator turning on to know what was coming next.

I now knew our reactions would be totally different, so I was able to go into listening to her being teased and begging for orgasm with my own erotic glee. By the time it was my turn, I was already close to getting off.

When everything was done, we collapsed into a snuggle pile on the bed and eventually got up the strength to make more cups of tea.

I wouldn't have been able to understand it if I hadn't been

part of it, but all my feelings of comparison and competition had melted away. It wasn't that we were interchangeable. What he got from playing with each of us was entirely different. And what each of us got out of it was different, too. I was deeply emotionally invested, and she was playfully having a good time.

I'd heard so much talk of threesomes causing jealousy, I couldn't believe a threesome had cured mine.[12]

Missing Communication

If there are problems in communication, they're going to show. You may think that once sex starts happening, it'll smooth over any issues, but usually the opposite is true. Sex will highlight any places where there's tension, missing communication, or fuzzy or crossed boundaries.

Take this example from Kat Stark, author of **Waking Up Polyamorous** *and* **Yelling In Pasties: The Wet Coast Confessions of an Anxious Slut:**

> *My worst threesome experiences have been to do with poor communication.*
>
> *In one example, I had traveled seven hours to visit a long-distance love, and I joined him and his partner in a threesome the first night I arrived. I was very attracted to her, and in normal circumstances I would want to get all up in her business, but the reality was I was really there for him. We hadn't seen each other in six months, and I wanted to focus on renewing that connection after a lengthy break, but I knew she tended to feel left out of things so I was hyper-conscious the entire time about making sure I was giving her as much attention as I could.*

---

12 Results not guaranteed.

Every time he and I began focusing on each other, the tension built in a really uncomfortable way, and I felt like we were doing something wrong. As the threesome went on, it became clearer and clearer that there was some sort of issue going on in their relationship that I wasn't privy to, and while each of us had had an orgasm by the end of the night, I don't think any of us left the experience feeling satisfied. We did not threesome again, and honestly, it killed my interest in group sex for quite a while.

If there's existing tension in your relationship, be sure to address it before adding people to the mix. And if you're noticing tension while you're playing, you're probably better off pausing for a conversation or rescheduling entirely, to avoid being turned off of group play for a long time.

Jealousy

To understand jealousy, we need to understand what we mean by the term. Jealousy is more of a category than a particular feeling of its own. And like any difficult feeling, it gives us information about our needs, wants, and boundaries.

Jealousy can be a catch-all term that includes feelings of comparison, envy, fear, insecurity, and much more. It's helpful to dig into exactly what you're feeling, because knowing what kind of jealousy you're experiencing is necessary for managing it.

Fear of jealousy is one of the main reasons I hear for avoiding threesomes, so it's worth exploring in detail. Hopefully you've done some exploration around this already, but let's dig a little deeper.

All the planning in the world can't prevent unexpected feelings from popping up in the moment. And while this might surprise you, it's *okay* to feel jealous.

Feeling jealous doesn't make you a bad partner or a bad friend or a bad lover. It doesn't even make you bad at threesomes. It just makes you human. You're the only one who can decide how distressing these feelings are and whether feeling them is a worthwhile price to pay to have the threesome experience you're considering.

Once you've decided to go ahead with the threesome, you'll need to keep checking in with yourself. Believe it or not, you may have to remind yourself to do this part. There's a lot going on in a threesome, and it's easy to get lost in the moment and not realize for a while that you're not entirely present.

Once you realize you're having a hard time with something, remember it's better to speak up in the moment than to do things you're not comfortable with or to stay in a situation you find upsetting. Continuing to push past your own boundaries can do you harm and can cause you to feel resentment towards the other people involved, and maybe towards threesomes in general.

Try to dig into what you're feeling in the moment—and what you need in response to that reaction. Then it's time to make a request.

Maybe what you need to ask for is that everything pause for a minute so you can get your bearings. Maybe there's a particular activity you need to stop or shift. If you have a partner in the mix, maybe you need a moment to check in with them or feel a little more connection.

It's always okay to ask for what you need—just keep in mind that if your request becomes a list of things you want the other people to do, it might be better to just call things to a halt.

If you're in a threesome with an existing partner, it can help to remember that you're in this together. This is an experience you've decided to share, and you're there as a team. So even if there's a moment when you're watching your partner do something with a new person and feeling left out, remember that it's still a shared experience. The threesome is what it is because you're there, too. Even if you don't feel entirely hands-on at every moment.

If you feel left out, ask yourself if the experience the other two are having is different because of you—and the answer is almost certainly yes. While people may seem distracted during sex, it's hard to forget you're being watched. And that means your presence is heightening the experience for everyone there, and likely increasing arousal too.

Remember that the experience you're sharing isn't just the sex. You've shared all the planning that went into making it happen, and you're going to have memories of the experience to share, too. You'll get to relive the threesome together, talk about your experience—from what you felt to what you saw—and you'll have dirty talk and arousal material to use for a long time going forward.

If you start to feel jealous, or left out, is there a way you can turn that around? Can you look at what's happening in front of you and find something to enjoy about what you're seeing? Can you imagine how you'll describe the scene to your partner later; what it was like watching them with another person? Jealousy and arousal are both such activated states that sometimes we can consciously shift from one to the other.

Crossed Boundaries

If you have enough threesomes (or really, enough sex of any kind), there's going to be a "whoops" at some point. Whether it's something silly, like someone tumbling out of the bed or taking an elbow to a sensitive spot, or something serious, like crossing a stated boundary, you'll need to respond.

Remember that people's boundaries and limits may not be intuitive to you. In fact, someone might dislike something that's a regular part of your sexual repertoire. I still feel bad about the time I licked someone's ear after they'd told me that was a limit for them. For some reason, it just didn't stick in my brain. We paused, I apologized, and they accepted my apology and felt okay to continue playing.

First of all, if you've crossed a boundary, take it seriously. It doesn't matter if you think it's a big deal—it matters how the other person feels. And acknowledging their feelings is key. In the moment, that might be tricky, because you may be embarrassed or even defensive. So do your best to move through those feelings and take care of the person who has been harmed.

Keep in mind the elements of a good apology. Take responsibility for what happened and acknowledge your actions. Make sure the other person knows you understand the situation. And if possible, share how you'll make sure it doesn't happen again.

Don't try to pass things off with, "I'm sorry you feel that way." And make sure you don't make excuses or try to diminish the severity of what happened. A bad apology only makes the situation worse.

What if you're the one whose boundary was crossed? First, you need to decide if you want to continue playing. If so, make sure the other people realize what has happened. Point out that a boundary was crossed, and restate your boundary, making sure everyone is clear. If there is understanding all around, and you're feeling comfortable, you might choose to resume playing.

And if it takes you totally out of the mood and you need to stop? That's okay too. It's still worth addressing in the moment, if you feel up to it. And then you can decide if you want to try again another time, or if you simply don't feel comfortable playing with this person or people again.

Treating People Like Merit Badges

Some people have a sexual bucket list, and if that leads to fun and adventure, then good for them! But it's important to remember that people are more than a tick-box on your list. So if some of your to-do list items slice and dice people by race, gender, or other physical identifiers, you might want to closely examine your motivations.

Think about the ways certain races, ethnicities, or bodies have been sexualized as part of their stereotyping. Considering certain people "exotic" is incredibly problematic, and falls under the category of treating people like objects or sexual props—one of the major threesome no-nos.

Black men, in particular, have been sexualized in a threesome context. While often part of a cuckolding fantasy, this fetishization can occur in any threesome dynamic. The fetishization of black men is so common in some sexual spaces that BBC (for big black cock) is a commonly understood acronym. Remember that reducing someone to a physical trait is demeaning and unethical.

A few years ago, as part of my advice column for my local newspaper, I did a piece about racism in threesome partner selection. For the piece, I reached out to several friends and colleagues for their insight. For this book, I talked to Kevin Patterson, author of *Love's Not Color Blind*, again. He echoed a lot of the themes that we've already discussed in this book, such as treating people with respect, while putting his own spin on the idea:

> *It's been my experience, as someone who has had a lot of threesomes, that the best sexy situations [are] when the people involved all respect one another. When the people involved all see one another. If you're looking at someone from a racially fetishized lens, you're not seeing this person, you're not respecting them—you're approaching them as*

just another object, as a dark-skinned dildo, in a situation that requires a full-fledged, well-rounded, respected human being.

You always have to do that mental math to make sure that's not the situation that you're in. If you're Black in America, you have to do that in every situation, but also in group sex situations.

If somebody is inviting you to a play party or to a threesome, and they don't know that much about you, you have to stop and wonder what is it that they know about you—what are they inviting, not who are they inviting.

Within the last couple of years, I've found myself among a group of friends who enjoy group sex. But where people know one another. We can have conversations, we can go out to eat, we can do other things, we can have our kids play together. But then we can also have group sex.

I've been in situations where I've felt like somebody was inviting me along who didn't really know me. Or someone would invite me to their home, but wouldn't invite me out with their friends. That's when you do the math in your head and say, "I know what's really happening here." And these are all well-meaning liberals, these are all people who would have voted for Obama for a third term, these are people who've seen Get Out in theaters.

I've been in situations where I'm having a conversation with somebody and talking about geek shit and they keep making it about race, or I'm talking about sports, and they're making it about race, and okay—I see what you think I bring to the table here. I see what perspective you're looking for.

It ends up being the math you have to do in so called sex-positive, group sex, orgy situations. You have to understand people are bypassing some of the typical getting-to-

know-you or vetting conversations, because they might feel they already know what they need for the activity they want you to engage in.

If you don't know me, and you feel like you know me, I know what it is that you think you know.

Everybody has their own measurement for . . . how much white nonsense they're willing to put up with. For me, I won't go to unfamiliar sexy places. I won't go to sexy places with unfamiliar hosts. I'm not going to take a partner and go to the local swing club. I'll go if I'm there with several people that I know. I'll go if it's a kink and queer night. I find that in those instances, the queer folks have a better understanding, having to deal with their own oppression. I find that kink spaces understand consent better. On those nights, I know I can do less mental math.

So I won't go places where I'm not familiar with the host, or where I'm not with a group of people, because if I get invited to fuck people I don't really know, I know they're not looking to fuck Kevin, I know they're looking for "big black cock." And that's not what I'm here for.

When it comes to choosing partners for threesomes or group sex, Kevin and I agree—it's better to get to know the person:

Ask yourself questions about the person you're trying to include in your sex. How much do you know about this person? Do you know their middle name? Do you know where they work? Do you know where they went to school? The things that round out a person. Do you know what their hopes and ambitions are? Do you know which way they vote? Do you know this person, or do you know about this person? Do you know who this person is, or do you know what this person is?

> *If you only know what they are, you should leave them alone.*

As for people who are just interested in casual sex?

> *Even if your goal is just to fuck, treating people like people makes that work better anyway. When you treat people well, you get to fuck again.*

For more great information from Kevin, check out his book, *Love's Not Color Blind*, especially the chapter about dating preferences.

FLEXIBILITY, IMPROVISATION, AND HAVING A PLAN B

Be Flexible

As we've discussed, you don't need to enact every fantasy you have during your first threesome. The more expectations you have, the more room there is for disappointment. Remember that if your threesome goes well, there's no reason there can't be a second, and a third, and so on. So better to keep it simple and have it go well (and leave everyone wanting more) than to try and do too much and feel disappointed.

Another reason to stay flexible is that it will help you enjoy the experience. If you're working your way through a mental threesome to-do list, you're not present in the moment, and you might realize later that you spent so much time choreographing that you forgot to enjoy yourself.

If you want to be ready for whatever comes, you've got a few options. You can have a whole list of positions and scenarios you want to try, while having no particular commitment to each one. That way you can easily switch from one suggestion to the next, depending on what feels good for everyone.

Or, you can challenge yourself to go into the bedroom with

no list at all, and simply go with the flow and see what the energy of the people manifests. (And if that's terrifying, you can always keep this book under the bed for reference if you feel stuck.)

Restrictions and Changes Are a Blessing

So, you get your dream threesome together and then find out someone has a boundary or limit you didn't know about—now what?

This might be a blessing in disguise.

Because you can't do exactly what you'd planned on, now you have to go with the flow and improvise in the moment. And that might lead to an even better experience than if things had gone as planned.

This is an experience I've had with rope bondage on more than one occasion. I'll make a rope date, and when we finally get down to playing, I'll learn something about my play partner's body that throws everything I'd planned out the window. In one example, I found out at the last minute that it wasn't good for my play partner to keep their knees bent for any length of time. So I had to entirely scrap my plans and just improvise. We ended up having an incredibly connective and sensual experience. Instead of the elaborate ties and positions I'd planned, we instead focused on the feeling of the rope as it moved across their skin and restrained their body. I watched their face and listened to the sounds they made and used that feedback as my guide for what to do next.

Had I not found out about a last-minute restriction, I would have moved through the series of poses I'd planned—and I would have had something to compare myself to. Would the ties I did look like the pictures I'd seen online? Or would it look like the time I'd seen it done at a party?

As long as there's an outside source to compare yourself to, it's easy to feel like you're falling short. But if you're simply enjoying the experience as it comes, it's impossible to do wrong.

MORE THAN A THREESOME?

Triads/Thrupples

Can what starts as a one-off threesome turn into a relationship? Absolutely. But it takes a lot of talking and a complete reconfiguration of the relationship. In an ethical triad, like in an ethical threesome, everybody's needs and feelings are considered. That means you can't simply tack a new person on to an existing relationship. Instead, you're forming a new relationship that involves three people.

Does that mean there can't be hierarchy in that new relationship? Not necessarily. But it's important that it's considered and negotiated, rather than the default setting based on seniority.

Typical structures for a triad are either a triangle where everyone is involved with everyone, or a *V* where there's a central person with two partners, but all three people are in the relationship, perhaps nesting together.

What gets tricky is if there's an imbalance in who can interact with whom. A triad is really four relationships. It's each person's relationship with each other person, and then the group as a whole.

Trying to legislate different levels within the triad can be tricky. For example, saying there can be threesomes, but the third can't have solo sex with either party—or can with one person but not the other. These kinds of rules can make trouble. They might work in the context of a one-off threesome, or even ongoing casual play partners, but in the context of a relationship it will likely spell disaster.

It's unrealistic to expect each wing of the relationship to have exactly the same depth and quality of feelings. If you're going to delve into this kind of relationship, you need to let each dynamic take its own shape.

Here's what Cooper Becket, author of My Life on the Swingset: Adventures in Swinging & Polyamory and A Life Less Monogamous has to say:

Hard to believe it's four years ago, already. At a party with some friends in January, my partner Elle and I met Taran. She "got" us, and we got her. We'd played together a couple of times, but mostly in bigger groups or as divided solo play. When we saw Taran at a party in March, something overwhelmed us a bit, and we all gravitated to each other. Despite the party having dozens of sexy people writhing and fucking all around us, our focus narrowed until it was only us three. That night we cycled through an ever rotating series of sexual combinations, tasting and feeling together, until we culminated in two variations of DP—first Elle wearing a harness and the two of us with Taran, and then Taran wearing it and the two of us fucking Elle. The experience blacked out the rest of the world, and even as the party wound down, we were just us three. That was the night we became a triad, and we celebrate it as our anniversary, even now, four years later.

Steady Play Partners

If a triad relationship sounds like too much work or too much negotiation, never fear, that's not the only way to keep the three-some action going with the same group of people.

While a triad can be a relationship that's both steady and serious, you can also have a relationship that's steady—or at least ongoing—while not being very serious.

There's a couple I've been seeing for threesomes for most of a year now, and it's still firmly in the casual category. They're married, they live together, and when we get together it's mostly for sex.

On our first date, we simply went out to dinner to get a sense of each other. We didn't go home together, we didn't so much as kiss. But there was enough chemistry and potential that our next date was dinner at my place, just in case. When we hit it off again, that second date led to sex. And the second date led to a third date, and so on.

But aside from our first dinner date, each subsequent date has been at my home. And while I cooked dinner the first time, the third date and beyond have been much simpler, usually just sharing dessert post sex. That's not to say our connection is only about sex. We sit and chat for a while before we get to that part, and we genuinely get along. We talk about our jobs and about current events, the way any friends would do. But at the same time, it's clear why they've come over.

Texting between dates is occasional. Maybe a sexy picture here and there or maybe a picture from a hike or a vacation. Just general check-ins. One of the ways you can make sure a connection stays in the casual realm is by not texting constantly. A few check-ins are nice, but if you're talking every day, that's the path to a more serious relationship.

★ ★ ★

There are a number of ways to form a steady or ongoing play partner arrangement. And luckily, they start the same way as finding a one-off threesome. Just like any first (or second) date that goes well, you check in the next day or a few days later and see if everyone would like to do it again sometime.

That doesn't mean "sometime" needs to be particularly soon. It can simply be on the table for the next time schedules align. And that can be a month, two months, or even more between dates.

This distance—both not talking constantly and not seeing a lot of each other—helps prevent more serious feelings from developing. So if you want ongoing without more serious commitment, just make sure your logistics are supporting that desire.

Swinging/Partner Swap

All of the considerations and negotiations for three people apply when playing with four or more—but more people, more problems? Not necessarily. Sometimes playing with even numbers of people, such as two couples, can feel easier because it's less likely to leave one odd person out.

At the same time, having two people pair off, like in a classic partner swap, can bring up unique issues. In a threesome, the idea is that all three people are playing together. With four or more, it's likely that little pairs or groups will form, so it's possible to feel less connected with an existing partner if you have one.

A classic swinging scenario is two couples (typically both M/F) who meet up and "swap" partners, often in the same space. The way this parallel play occurs is usually within sight of the other folks playing, but while you've also got your hands full. So you've got the support of your partner there, and some voyeurism and exhibitionism action, while being busy enough that you're not watching every single thing the other people are doing.

One of the tricks here is making sure each pair is equally

enthusiastic about the trade off. You don't want to get stuck with someone feeling like they need to "take one for the team" because their partner is excited about it. Again, we never want someone having sex they're not fully on board with. So if you're going this route, take the time to find people you both really feel good about.

Group Sex

Where does something make the jump to group sex? I think it depends on the configuration as much as it does on the number of people. With four people, you can have a partner swap or a group experience. Once you hit five people, you're looking at a higher likelihood of breakout groups.

Here are some examples from my life:

I was in a foursome scenario that didn't include any preexisting couples. There was a fella I'd been on some dates with, but we didn't operate as a couple. More like kink play partners. One evening I met up with him and two of his other friends, one I knew and one I didn't. Both were women. The four of us were getting together to go to a polyamory meetup together. After the event, we all went back to the fella's house.

Spoiler alert: we all ended up having sex together. And this was one of those situations that could be described as organic or spontaneous—at least by an outside observer—because we didn't get together for the purpose of sex, and there wasn't a whole lot of conversation in advance.

But I think of it as a situation with hidden preparation, rather than being truly spontaneous. All four of us were already "orgy people." We were variously active in sex-positive, kink, and poly communities, and all of us had great communication skills plus experience with multiperson sex.

This is why I stress the importance of becoming the kind of

person that group sex or threesomes happen to. There's groundwork you can do well in advance.

The four of us snuggled on the couch for a while, and eventually there was some kissing. Before any particular pair kissed, someone always asked permission. This is one of the many ways you can demonstrate that you're good at communication, and put people at ease with good consent practices. Because we were asking about everything from the very beginning, from kissing, to where we put our hands, to eventually taking clothes off, everyone knew that nothing would happen before we were ready for it.

Eventually the couch became too awkward for four bodies and someone proposed a move to the bed. We all went and fell back into a pile. As is often the case with groups of four, we paired off a bit. I began going down on one of the women, while the fella bent the other woman over the bed to penetrate her from behind. So while we weren't all involved in the exact same sex acts, we all had a great view of what was going on.

Over the course of the evening, people swapped around and tried different things. The fella and I had an existing agreement that we didn't engage in penetrative sex together, so during this group play that simply didn't come up. That's another example of how having standing agreements can make things move more smoothly when you find yourself in group play.

That particular combination of people never got together for sex again, but everyone is still friends to this day.

What about the line between group sex and a sex party? More than five? More than seven?

I had an experience with six people that you could call a small sex party. It consisted of my then triad (myself plus one man and one woman), two women who were girlfriends, and an AMAB[13] nonbinary person.

This particular group was all made up of friends and acquaintances, but not everyone in the group had been sexual with each other before. And within the group there were different degrees of both friendship and attraction.

We all got together with the explicit understanding that this was a sex party. But we eased into things slowly. We had dinner together and shared a lot of small talk before taking things even further.

In advance of the gathering, we prepared a space. We knew that six people would be too many for the queen-sized bed, so instead we brought a futon mattress and placed it on the living room floor, in front of the couch. A few sheets and blankets later, and we had a great cuddle zone.

This set-up was useful because it was easy to transition from kissing on the couch to rolling around on the (padded) floor. And it offered enough space for any combination of people— whether the whole group wanted to engage at once, or whether pairs or threesomes wanted to break off.

Having so many people meant a lot of options. It also made it easy for one or two people to take a snack break or get something to drink while other people were still playing. With more bodies it can be easier to slide in or out of the mix without being disruptive.

There was no PIV sex during this encounter. But there was lots of making out, hand sex, fisting, and prostate stimulation with both fingers and toys.

We also skipped oral sex, which meant that it was easier to maintain boundaries between people who didn't want to swap fluids. We simply swapped gloves between activities and between

---

13 Assigned Male At Birth

partners and always knew that was keeping people safe. Everyone was kissing everyone, so by keeping genital fluids off our mouths, we never had to remember who had been where, or run to the bathroom to wash our mouths or faces between activities.

If you can think beyond PIV or oral sex, there are tons of options and combinations of sex to be had—and you may find that the whole encounter can last even longer when you're thinking outside the box.

24

AFTERCARE

What Is Aftercare?

In the kink and BDSM world, *aftercare* is the term used for the cool-down period after a scene. When we've experienced a period of intensity, whether physical or emotional, we can be left in a vulnerable state. Sometimes we're not even aware of what we need in the moment, so it's a great idea to plan ahead.

Aftercare often includes being wrapped up in a blanket, having some water and a snack, and sharing some snuggles.

If you think about it, you likely already have an aftercare routine for your sex. Do you snuggle? Shower together? Get a drink of water? Share some pillow talk?

Whatever you usually do, think about doing it with three. No one wants to be rushed out of bed after sex. And while there doesn't need to be an overnight (depending on what you've negotiated), at least let everyone catch their breath and feel good about the adventure before going their separate ways.

The kind of aftercare you do will be the lasting impression people head out the door with, or go to sleep thinking about, and aftercare routine can make or break whether there's a second threesome with the same group of people.

Check-Ins with All Parties

Even if you've done sweet aftercare right after your threesome, it's a good idea to have at least one follow up in the days to come, unless there's a specific agreement not to.

Simply sending a text the next day is a nice gesture, and it opens the door for communication if there are issues to be discussed. Mostly it's a nice way for everyone to say a quick thank you and reinforce a good feeling about the encounter.

Especially if you think you'd like to get the same combination of people together again sometime, it's much easier to text a proposition in a couple of weeks or months if you've already sent a nice message that wasn't asking for something.

If you'd like to have a repeat performance, it's a good idea to have a chat about what went well and what could be improved next time. This chat can happen in the days following the threesome, or it can be part of the negotiation for next time. In fact, even if you're not going to do it again, it can be helpful to discuss highlights and lowlights, so your next sexual encounter can benefit from that information, even if it's with different people.

If someone was the center of attention for most of the threesome, it could be nice to plan a different focus for the next time, so that everyone can share in the benefits of multiperson sex. That can also be a useful and flirtatious thing to text. Maybe telling someone that you're excited for them to be the star of the show next time, or mentioning something you'd love to do with them. It doesn't hurt to start building anticipation, even if it'll be a while before you get together.

Post-Threesome Dates

A great way to reinforce the idea that no one in the threesome is just a plaything is to go on a nonsexual date after the threesome has happened. This way you're building connection that can support future play, or simply solidifying a friendship if play was a one-off.

If the threesome involves people who were already friends but hadn't had sex before, a post-threesome get-together can smooth the transition back into friendly hang-outs, and prove sooner rather than later that everyone can still get along outside of the bedroom.

If your threesome led to an overnight, going out to brunch the next day is an excellent option. If everyone went their separate ways, or has work first thing in the morning, consider scheduling a hangout soon, if this is the dynamic you're hoping to create.

Reconnection Time If There's an Existing Couple

When an existing couple has an encounter with a third, it can be nice to plan some reconnection time in advance. Perhaps the partners spend the night together and the third goes home. Or, if everyone is staying over, maybe the reconnection is over coffee or breakfast the next day, or a date in the next day or two. Try to do it sooner rather than later, so that no difficult feelings have time to fester. Even the most confident among us likes to hear some sweetness from our partner after watching them have sex with someone else.

I actually had to explain this to a partner once. The day after a threesome, I told him I could use some sweetness and reassurance, and he was completely surprised. He told me that I seemed so confident that he hadn't even imagined that was something I'd need. And then he proceeded to give me the reassurance I needed. While it's lovely to hear that I present as so confident, it's a good reminder that everyone likes some reassurance now and then.

Conversations that can be valuable include discussing what was fun about sharing this experience with your partner, what you learned by watching them with someone else, and what was especially hot.

It's helpful to celebrate the things that were fun, or that went well, to reinforce feeling good about the experience. Even if some areas need improvement, don't forget to also discuss the good parts, so you're not completely soured on threesomes going forward.

What were the highlights? What hot images are stuck in your head? Reliving these memories can propel fantasy and dirty talk for weeks, months, or years going forward.

Remember, though, that when talking about a threesome after the fact, you still want to be sensitive to any insecurities you discussed going into the threesome. Just because the actual threesome is over, the same guidelines apply. Don't fall into comparison talk or anything else that is likely to hurt feelings.

One caveat: whatever reconnection you're planning, make sure it doesn't come at the expense of the feelings of your third. For example, if you want the third to go home so the established couple can spend the night together, make sure that's negotiated in advance, and something everyone feels good about. Don't simply throw them out as soon as sex is over.

Be Gentle with Yourself

There's a bit of advice I often give my clients at the end of a session: if at any point this process feels like work, or you find yourself dreading any part of it, it may be time to take a break. Sure, there can be a bit of discomfort when we're trying new things, but make sure you're not pushing yourself too far, too fast.

We're aiming for fun and adventure, for intimacy and growth. And those things aren't achieved in any one way. Hopefully, we spend our whole lives learning and trying new things. So there's no rush to have a threesome, or any other sexual experience.

Keep an open mind.
Try new things.
Have fun.

GLOSSARY

AFAB—Assigned female at birth.

AMAB—Assigned male at birth.

Barrier—Any form of physical safer sex protection, like a condom or dental dam.

BDSM—Bondage, Discipline, Dominance, Submission, Sadism, Masochism.

Bisexual— someone who identifies as bisexual is attracted to people of both their same gender and people of different genders.

Cisgender—A person whose gender identity aligns with the gender they were assigned at birth.

Compersion—feeling joy for your partner's joy.

Cuckold—A person who enjoys watching or hearing about their partner's sexual experience with someone else. Usually in reference to a man.

Cuckqueen—A person who enjoys watching or hearing about their partner's sexual experience with someone else. Usually in reference to a woman.

Dental dam—A safer-sex barrier that consists of a rectangle of latex (or other material) that prevents fluid exchange or skin-to-skin contact during oral sex on a vulva or anus.

Devil's threesome—a threesome that includes two men and one woman. The term comes from the "devil horns" hand gesture you see at rock concerts, where in this case each horn is a penis.

Dominant/submissive—A power exchange in a kink or BDSM context. For the space of the scene (or the relationship), the submissive gives power to the dominant.

Dyad—any pair of people. In this context it's used to distinguish between a romantic couple and a pair of friends who may engage as a unit during a threesome, or may come to the threesome as an existing unit.

Ethical nonmonogamy—an umbrella term for a variety of consensual nonmonogamous relationships. Meant to distinguish from unethical nonmonogamy, aka cheating.

Femme—Having your gender presentation be feminine. Often as part of a queer identity.

Fluid bonded—a term used in polyamory to describe a couple who doesn't use any barriers during sex. This means they share fluids during oral and/or penetrative sex.

FMF, MFM, FFM, MMF—various shorthand terms for a threesome, where the M and F stand for Male and Female. The positions of the letters are sometimes used to indicate what level of involvement each person would have (i.e. an MFM might be a spit-roast situation where the men don't touch each other), but also sometimes used interchangeably.

Full swap—A term typically used in swinging, when two couples come together and "swap" partners. Often this is done as parallel play, in the same room.

GGG - Good, Giving, and Game, a term coined by Dan Savage that you may run into on dating sites. Used to indicate that the person is sex-positive, maybe a little kinky, and generally open-minded.

Heteroflexible—Someone who is primarily attracted to people of another gender but who is "flexible" in certain play scenarios.

Homoflexible—Someone who is primarily attracted to people of the same gender but who is "flexible" in certain play scenarios.

Internal condom—A prophylactic device meant to be worn by the receiver of penetration. Can be used in a vaginal canal or rectum. (Most commonly sold under the brand FC2.)

Kink—A colloquial term for BDSM, often referring to anything that's a bit edgy or alternative in the sexual realm.

Nesting–Partners who live together, sometimes used to avoid more hierarchical language.

Nonbinary (enby)—Someone whose gender identity is neither male nor female, and who also rejects the idea of gender as a binary.

Pansexual—Someone attracted to people of all genders.

Parallel play—Often in a swinging context, engaging in sexual play in view of other people, but without crossover of activities.

Pegasus—A male unicorn, meaning a single man who joins a M/F couple for a threesome.

Pickup play—A term used in the kink and BDSM scene (though potentially relevant to sex parties as well) where players meet at the party and pick each other up, rather than having had plans in advance, or a preexisting relationship.

PIV—Penis in vagina.

Play partner—Used in the kink scene to refer to someone you engage in kink play with, and used more generally as someone you may have casual sexual encounters with.

Polyamory—Literally, "many loves." Polyamory refers to a relationship structure where people engage in multiple relationships with the knowledge and consent of all parties.

Polyfidelity—A polyamorous relationship that is open within the group, but not open to outsiders. Could refer to a triad/thrupple or even a whole community.

Relationship anarchy—Applying the principles of anarchy to relationships. People who are relationship anarchists generally practice nonhierarchy and value personal autonomy.

Strap-on—A harness that fits around the waist and thighs to

attach a dildo to the wearer in a way that's sturdy enough for penetration in a variety of positions.

Soft swap—a term from swinging that describes two couples playing together in a way that includes hand sex and oral sex, but not PIV.

Solo-polyamory—a form of polyamory where someone has no primary partner, but maintains multiple relationships.

Swinging/Swinger—People who engage in partner sharing or swapping.

Thrupple—A newer term for triad.

Top/bottom—Often heard in the queer or kink scenes, top refers to the person giving or doing, and bottom refers to the person receiving. For example: in a spanking, the top is doing the spanking and the bottom is receiving the spanking.

Triad—A relationship between three people. Can refer to a relationship where everyone is involved with everyone, or a *V* relationship, where two people are dating the central "hinge" of the *V*, but not each other.

Unicorn—Generally, any third in a threesome scenario. Initially coined to refer to an attractive bisexual woman who would join a couple to fulfill their fantasies while not having needs of her own, and who would then go her own way. Termed unicorn because such people don't exist.

Unicorn hunters—a somewhat derogatory term applied to couples who seek a unicorn for a threesome. Frowned upon because of the tendency of some couples to treat the third as an object.

RESOURCES

Dating apps and websites come and go almost too quickly to put in print, so use this list to start exploring, but be ready to browse an app store or the latest online advice to see what spaces on the internet have a critical mass when you're looking.

Dating apps:

Hinge, for general dating

#open, an app aimed at people interested in open relationships

Feeld, an app for individuals and couples looking for threesomes, open relationships, or kink

Adult FriendFinder, a website for people looking for more casual partners

Tinder, for general dating or hookups

OkCupid, for general dating, for singles or couples

Bumble, for general dating

HER, a dating app for women

Websites/social networks/communities:

Scarleteen: wonderful information about sex, consent, and communication

FetLife: a kink and BDSM social media site

Kasidie: a swingers social media site

Reddit: there are subreddits on everything from open relationships to BDSM to even threesomes

Hey Epiphora: sex toy reviews

Poly Role Models: a blog about polyamory

Podcasts:

Life on the Swingset

Polyamory Weekly

Savage Lovecast

Speaking of Sex with the Pleasure Mechanics

Sex Gets Real with Dawn Serra

American Sex Podcast

Sex Out Loud

Shameless Sex

Girl Boner Radio with August McLaughlin

Multiamory

Books:

Tongue Tied: Untangling Communication in Sex, Kink, and Relationships by Stella Harris

As Kinky as You Wanna Be: Your Guide to Safe, Sane and Smart BDSM by Shanna Germain

The Ethical Slut: A Practical Guide to Polyamory, Open Relationships & Other Adventures by Janet W. Hardy and Dossie Easton

Love's Not Color Blind: Race and Representation in Polyamorous and Other Alternative Communities by Kevin Patterson

She Comes First: The Thinking Man's Guide to Pleasuring a Woman by Ian Kerner

Come As You Are: The Surprising New Science that Will Transform Your Sex Life by Emily Nagoski

Redefining Our Relationships: Guidelines For Responsible Open Relationships by Wendy-O Matik

Girl Sex 101 by Allison Moon and kd diamond

Three-Way: Erotic Stories by Alison Tyler

Online shopping options:

SheVibe Pleasure Boutique

Good Vibrations

She Bop

Tantus

Funkit Toys

Switch Leather Co.

InHerTube

JoEllen Notte maintains a "superhero sex shops" list that can help you find a store near you.

THREESOME YES/NO/MAYBE LIST

Flirting

Kissing

Cuddling

Undressing

Hand sex (giving)

Hand sex (receiving)

Oral sex (giving)

Oral sex (receiving)

Vaginal sex (giving)

Vaginal sex (receiving)

Anal sex (giving)

Anal sex (receiving)

Bondage

Spanking

Overnights

Using sex toys

Watching porn together

Sex in your home/bed

Sex with friends

Sex with coworkers

Sex with exes

Seeing a threesome partner solo (i.e., meet as a couple and then have individual dates)

Sex with other couples

ENDNOTES

i   Clapham, Phil, Peter Duley, Barbara Lagerquist, Bruce Mate, Alison Stimpert, Frederick Wenzel. "Observations of a Female North Atlantic Right Whale (Eubalaena glacialis) in Simultaneous Copulation with Two Males: Supporting Evidence for Sperm Competition," *Aquatic Mammals* 31 (2005): 157–160. doi:10.1578/AM.31.2.2005.157.

ii Lehmiller, Justin, *Tell Me What You Want: The Science of Sexual Desire and How It Can Help You Improve Your Sex Life.* Hachette Book Group, 2018.

iii Kilgallon, Sarah J and Leigh W Simmons. "Image content influences men's semen quality" *Biology Letters* 1 (2005): 253–255. http://doi.org/10.1098/rsbl.2005.0324.

iv Meston, Cindy M, and David M Buss. "Why humans have sex," *Archives of Sexual Behavior* 36, no. 4 (2007): 477–507. doi:10.1007/s10508-007-9175-2. https://pubmed.ncbi.nlm.nih.gov/17610060/.

v   O'Malley, Harris. "Ask Dr. NerdLove: The Rule of Threesomes." Paging Dr. Nerdlove, March 21, 2012. https://www.doctornerdlove.com/dr-nerdlove-rule-threesomes/.

vi Bailey, Michael J, Meredith L Chivers, Gerulf Rieger, and Ritch C Savin-Williams. "Sexual arousal and masculinity-femininity of women," *Journal of Personality and Social Psychology* 111, no. 2 (2016): 265–283. doi:10.1037/pspp0000077. https://pubmed.ncbi.nlm.nih.gov/26501187/.

vii To read more about the methodology problems, read "The Problem with Sexual Arousal Studies" by Alice Dreger, as published in *Pacific*

Standard: https://psmag.com/social-justice/problem-sexual-arousal-studies-87383.

viii Copen, Casey E., Anjani Chandra, and Isaedmarie Febo-Vazquez. "Sexual Behavior, Sexual Attraction, and Sexual Orientation Among Adults Aged 18–44 in the United States: Data From the 2011–2013 National Survey of Family Growth," *National Health Statistics Reports* 88 (January 7, 2016). http://i2.cdn.turner.com/cnn/2016/images/01/06/nhsr88.pdf.

ix Carrillo, Héctor, and Amanda Hoffman. "'Straight with a Pinch of Bi': The Construction of Heterosexuality as an Elastic Category among Adult US Men." *Sexualities* 21, no. 1–2 (2017): 90–108. https://doi.org/10.1177/1363460716678561.

x Bruce Kirschbaum and Sam Kass, "The Switch," *Seinfeld*, season 6, episode 11, directed by Andy Ackerman, aired January 5, 1995. NBC.

xi Brown, Kara. "The Problem With Calling Women 'Females'." Jezebel, February 5, 2015. https://jezebel.com/the-problem-with-calling-women-females-1683808274.

xii Clayton, Tracy, and Heben Nigatu. "6 Reasons You Should Stop Referring To Women As 'Females' Right Now." BuzzFeed. https://www.buzzfeed.com/tracyclayton/stop-calling-women-females.